Mothers surviving chil

A common reaction when people think themselves into the shoes of women whose children have been sexually abused by their partners or anyone else is to say instantly 'I'd kill them'. It is an attempt to deflect pain with a simple remedy, but faced with the reality women's reactions are considerably more complex. The central aim of *Mothers Surviving Child Sexual Abuse* is to demonstrate this complexity, and to explore the way it is embedded in the social relations within which child sexual abuse takes place.

Using in-depth interviews with women whose children have been sexually abused, Carol-Ann Hooper investigates how they experience and cope with the situation and the difficulties they face. How do they find out that sexual abuse, nearly always surrounded in secrecy, has occurred? How do they decide what action to take? How do they experience the responses of others – friends, family, professionals? And how do they cope with their own feelings? The answers to such questions are crucial both to the children's safety and well-being, and to successful professional intervention.

Mothers Surviving Child Sexual Abuse offers a new analysis of mothers' reactions and responses and presents a fresh perspective on a difficult problem. Informed by theory and research on other situations involving loss, secrecy and moral dilemmas, as well as the rapidly accumulating knowledge of child sexual abuse, the book will be immensely helpful to practitioners and policy-makers involved in child protection, as well as to students and teachers in Social Work, Social Policy and Women's Studies.

Carol-Ann Hooper is Lecturer in Social Policy at the University of York.

Mothers surviving child sexual abuse

Carol-Ann Hooper

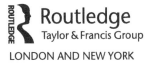

Routledge
Taylor & Francis Group

LONDON AND NEW YORK

First published 1992
by Routledge

2 Park Square, Milton Park, Abingdon, Oxon OX14 4RN
711 Third Avenue, New York, NY 10017, USA

Routledge is an imprint of the Taylor & Francis Group, an informa business

First issued in paperback 2016

Transferred to Digital Printing 2007

Typeset in Times by LaserScript Limited, Mitcham, Surrey

British Library Cataloguing in Publication Data
A catalogue record for this book is available from the British Library.

Library of Congress Cataloging in Publication Data

Hooper, Carol-Ann, 1956–
  Mothers surviving child sexual abuse/Carol-Ann Hooper.
  p. cm.
  Includes bibliographical references and index.
  1. Sexually abused children – United States – Family relationships – Case studies. 2. Incest victims – United States – Family relationships – Case studies. 3. Mothers – United States – Attitudes – Case studies.
  HV6570.7.H66   1992
  362.7'63'0973–dc20   92-7607
                                                                   CIP
ISBN 978-0-415-07187-1 (hbk)
ISBN 978-1-138-99423-2 (pbk)

Publisher's Note
The publisher has gone to great lengths to ensure the quality of this reprint but points out that some imperfections in the original may be apparent

Contents

Acknowledgements

I would like to thank first and foremost the fifteen women who volunteered to be interviewed for the study, and who took time and trouble to talk at length about personal and painful aspects of their lives. I hope the book achieves some of their hopes for it. I am grateful also to the Social Services Departments who cooperated in helping me to contact women whose children had been sexually abused, to the department which gave me access to its files and to the individual social workers who took precious time out from other demands to discuss their work with me.

I am indebted also to many others who have helped in various ways, with encouragement, critical comments and practical help. The Economic and Social Research Council provided funding for three years under the Postgraduate Studentship Scheme. Jane Lewis gave extensive advice throughout the research process and I am especially grateful to her. I thank also Bob Coles, Tony Fowles, Liz Gifford, Tony Hooper, Liz Kelly, Amy Manchershaw, Laura Markowe, Vivien Nice, Jennifer Peck, Janice Peggs, Catherine Rees and Jane Ribbens for their contributions.

Introduction

A common reaction when people think themselves into the shoes of a woman whose child has been sexually abused, by her partner or anyone else, is to say instantly 'I'd kill him'. It is both an attempt to deflect pain with a simple remedy and a reflection of the dominant contemporary discourse of motherhood, in which mothering is constructed as a matter of natural, unproblematic, instinctive response to children's needs for protection. Faced with the reality, women's reactions are considerably more complex – fortunately for those (mostly men and boys) who sexually abuse children, and also for children who are abused whose difficulties would certainly be compounded by the prosecution and probable imprisonment of their mothers. The central aim of this book is to demonstrate the complexity of mothers' responses and the way they are embedded in the social relations within which child sexual abuse occurs.

As recognition of child sexual abuse and professional experience have grown during the last decade, so has awareness of the complex dilemmas it raises for all those paid for their involvement in child protection work. Professional experts have acquired greater humility in the face of their own failures and mistakes. In the mainstream professional literature, such understanding has rarely been extended to the women on whose unpaid care both workers and children rely in the aftermath of abuse. The mother-blaming in much of this literature has been identified by previous feminist work (Nelson, 1987; Hooper, 1987; MacLeod and Saraga, 1988). The secondary aim of this book is to contribute to more realistic expectations of and appropriate help for mothers, and hence also for children who are sexually abused.

The book is based primarily on a study involving depth interviews with fifteen women whose children had been sexually abused. It is a small sample on which to base a book. However, the women's accounts were complex and detailed, and the aim of providing an initial exploration of a neglected area I hope justifies the sample size. The study was informed by a feminist perspective, by which I mean it aimed to make women's experience visible and to ground analysis in their own accounts. By and large, feminist theory on child sexual abuse has taken the accounts of adult women survivors as its starting point. Extending this to include the experiences of mothers, while recognising both the interconnectedness and the potential conflict between women and their children, is a necessary complement.

The book also draws in parts on a small study of social work cases of child sexual abuse, in which thirteen case records were analysed and the social workers interviewed to explore 'the other side' of the mother–social worker interaction. That study is written up elsewhere (Hooper, 1990), but I draw on its analysis here to identify parallels between the responses of mothers and of social workers, and in considering the implications of the main study for social work practice. There is increasing recognition of the importance of their mothers' support for children who are sexually abused, so that working with mothers to enable them to support their children has become a central task for workers involved in child protection. Mothers and workers are not clearly separate groups of course. During the time I was conducting the research I met women social workers and child abuse researchers who had suspected or discovered that their own children had been sexually abused, with similar consequences for them to those described by the women I interviewed. This overlap is often unrecognised in the professional construction of clients as an other, and by implication problem, group.

The book's title is intended to represent the sense women expressed of their active struggles in response to the threats they had experienced (from the abuse itself, and from the reactions of others). In work on violence against women and children, feminists have recently replaced the term 'victim' with 'survivor', to overcome the association of the former with passivity and with the study of victimology. Neither is particularly satisfactory, if they are taken to imply whole identities. Victimisation is a process, as is survival, and they may (or may not) coexist. The agent of the first is the perpetrator of violence, the agent of the second the woman or child victimised. There is a danger in this shift of labels of losing sight of the reality of violence. Not all women do survive it. This is no less true of sexual abuse than of other forms of violence, although the risk of death lies more in suicide than in murder. There is also a danger of flattening out all responses to the same level – survival should, after all, be a minimal aim. Nevertheless, women whose children have been sexually abused have claimed the label of survivors for themselves in recognition of both their suffering and their strength (Baghramian and Kershaw, 1989).

It is common in the mainstream literature to refer to women in this position only as 'mothers' (and sometimes to reduce them further to 'maternal responses') and to men who abuse as 'perpetrators'. I have tried where possible to avoid this, to recognise in language that all those involved, women, children and men who abuse have whole lives, identities and biographies. Sexual abuse is only one part of these, however important a one, and its meaning for each individual is constructed partly by this broader context of ongoing life histories.

1   Child sexual abuse and mothers

The issues

The sexual abuse of children has been a consistently high-profile public issue throughout the late 1980s, and continues to be one. It is not a new problem, nor is this the first period of its recognition. That it was adult survivors speaking out in the 1970s about their childhood experiences which initiated the current period of concern demonstrates that the problem itself is a long-standing one, and this is confirmed – at least for the USA – by research which has addressed the question of historical trends in incidence. In the UK, the public silence which preceded the current anxiety was itself preceded by a period of roughly sixty years, from the 1870s to the 1930s, of social anxiety and campaigns for more effective action to prevent the sexual abuse of children.[1]

Through this history of fluctuating visibility, the problem has been defined in various ways, reflecting the relative power of the different interest groups and social movements involved in promoting the issue. Children and women have relatively little power over such definitions, and they have often been blamed for the abuse perpetrated by men. Both the responses of voluntary and statutory agencies and the theories of academics and clinicians demonstrate this. In the responses of agencies, the surveillance of girls and their mothers has played a more prominent part than the control of men who abuse. The main focus has shifted from the surveillance of sexually abused girls in the early part of this century towards the surveillance of the mothers of sexually abused children in the later part. Theoretical explanations followed a similar trend. In the 1930s, the dominant explanation of incest, influenced by psychoanalytic ideas, focused on girls seducing their fathers (cf. Bender and Blau, 1937; Sloane and Karpinski, 1942). During the 1950s and 1960s this was gradually replaced by the dysfunctional or pathological family analysis which accorded mothers the central 'role' in father–daughter incest (cf. Kaufman *et al.*, 1954; Lustig *et al.*, 1966).

Feminists, who have played an important part in achieving public recognition in both the earlier period of concern and the later, have attempted to counter such definitions, locating child sexual abuse within the broader problem of men's violence against women and children and in its context in a male-dominated society. Patterns of violence tend to reflect and reinforce existing power relations, and child sexual abuse is no exception. Men are most likely to be the abusers, and girls are more likely than boys to be sexually abused. Father–daughter incest is not a wholly aberrant deviation, but an expression of the normal power relations of gender and age in families in a patriarchal society, albeit in extreme form. Feminist attempts to redefine the problem of child sexual abuse – from a family problem to a problem primarily of masculinity – have had some success in recent years. This redefinition has not occurred without conflict however, and the role of mothers in relation to child sexual abuse continues to be both controversial and crucial for children and professionals.

This chapter gives, first, an analysis of the role of mothers in relation to child sexual abuse, drawing on available research. It then discusses briefly the theoretical debate between 'family dysfunction' (or family systems) and feminist perspectives – offering a framework for the key contested issues of explanation and responsibility – and considers the implications of the current policy context for women whose children are sexually abused. Finally, it sets out the approach taken in the study on which this book is based.

CHILD SEXUAL ABUSE AND CHILD PROTECTION: THE ROLE OF MOTHERS

In policy documents and in the professional literature, child abuse is commonly associated with parents (the problem) and child protection with professionals (the solution). This is not unproblematic for any form of child abuse, since parents are not indivisible – one parent may protect the child from abuse by the other – and professionals cannot guarantee to improve matters for children.[2] It is particularly problematic however in relation to child sexual abuse. Neither the patterns of sexual abuse itself nor those of the protection of children in the aftermath fit at all comfortably onto this map.

The vast majority of incidents of child sexual abuse are not perpetrated by parents. The most recent UK study of prevalence (Kelly *et al.*, 1991) found 1 per cent of respondents reported sexual abuse by a parent (father or stepfather), compared with 47 per cent of the whole sample reporting some form of sexually intrusive experience before the age of 18 (59 per cent of young women and 27 per cent of young men).[3] While state intervention tends to focus primarily on intrafamilial abuse, the majority of experiences of sexual abuse are perpetrated not by close relatives nor by strangers, but by known adults (including more distant relatives) or peers.

Where sexual abuse is perpetrated by a parent or parent substitute, it is rarely the child's mother. Sexual abuse is predominantly committed by men – 85 per cent of abuse by peers and 95 per cent of abuse by adults (Kelly *et al.*, 1991). While mothers who sexually abuse their children do exist, they accounted for none of 1,051 incidents in the same study. This study may well have underestimated abuse by parents since respondents, aged 16–21, may have been reluctant to reveal abuse by those on whom they still depended. Russell's American study, based on women only but including a broader age range, found a higher rate of abuse by fathers or father substitutes (4.5 per cent), but still only 0.1 per cent reported abuse by mothers or mother substitutes (Russell, 1984). Since boys are more likely than girls to be abused by women, this is probably also an underestimate of sexual abuse by mothers. However, since boys are less likely than girls to be abused at all, it is clear that amongst parents who sexually abuse, men far outnumber women. Since child sexual abuse commonly occurs in secret, with only the abuser and child present, and mothers cannot therefore be assumed to know of abuse by others, mothers are non-abusing parents in all but a tiny minority of incidents, whether the perpetrator is within or outside the home.

The secrecy which surrounds child sexual abuse means the possibility of protection relies a great deal on children telling someone. Incidents of child sexual abuse which come to the attention of agencies comprise a small minority of the total – about 5 per cent (Russell, 1984; Kelly *et al.*, 1991). In Kelly *et al.*'s study, nearly half of those who experienced abuse had, however, told someone at the time. Children are often ambivalent about telling anyone. When they do, the majority of girls tell female friends or relatives (Manchershaw, 1987; Kelly *et al.*, 1991). Boys are less likely than girls to tell anyone, and more likely when they do to tell male friends or relatives. The bulk of the work of child protection is done not by professionals but by children themselves, their friends and parents.

To a large extent, while sexual abuse is perpetrated predominantly by men, the protection of children in the aftermath falls mainly to women. In Kelly *et al.*'s study, mothers were told of a higher number of incidents than were agencies, and female friends or sisters of a higher number still. While female friends or sisters were told of more assaults overall, mothers were more likely to be told where the girl was abused by an adult, and female peers where the abuser was under 18. This suggests that the less girls are able to protect themselves, the more they turn to mothers rather than peers. For those children who do not tell or whose abuse is not detected at the time, telling their mothers often remains an important issue in their recovery, years or decades later (Schatzow and Herman, 1989).

In the context of child sexual abuse, mothers can be said to be the primary adult actors in child protection. They are more likely than professionals to be told of abuse. Where professionals do become involved, the decision as to whether to remove children from home depends crucially on the ability and willingness of their mothers to protect them from further contact with the abuser. One study of such decisions found the mother's belief and cooperation with agencies the two most significant factors, more important than the severity or frequency of abuse (Pellegrin and Wagner, 1990). Their mothers' responses are also one of the key factors in children's recovery. Support from a non-abusing mother is one of if not the most significant factor(s) in uncoupling abuse from both short-term and long-term effects (Wyatt and Mickey, 1987; Conte and Berliner, 1988; Everson *et al.*, 1989; Gomes-Schwartz *et al.*, 1990).

Not all women whose children are sexually abused by others do respond supportively, although it is the minority, and possibly a shrinking minority, who do not. All studies conducted so far of mothers' responses to abuse by others – all in the USA – have found a majority being supportive or protective to the child. The figures range from 56 per cent of mothers being judged protective in a sample of children abused by fathers/father substitutes (Myer, 1984) to 80 per cent of mothers having taken some form of protective action and 90 per cent showing at least a moderate degree of concern for the child in a sample of children abused by family members and others (Gomes-Schwartz *et al.*, 1990).[4] Looking at the studies in chronological order, it appears that the proportion of mothers responding supportively may be increasing. Studies are not easily comparable since they define their samples and outcomes differently, and the trend is not wholly consistent. But it is likely that increased public awareness of child sexual abuse and more sympathetic agency responses to mothers have influenced mothers' responses.

Most studies of mothers' responses have sought factors which distinguish protective from non-protective mothers, with fairly limited success. The limitations of the research are in part those of the researchers' theoretical frameworks. Informed for the most part by psychological perspectives, studies more commonly examine the significance of women's own experiences of abuse in childhood than, for example, their current economic status or social support. Studies are further limited by their samples and methodological difficulties. Their samples are cases reported to agencies – a small minority of all incidents and one in which working-class families are overrepresented. It is generally more difficult to collect information from women who deny the abuse long term, reject the child or drop out of treatment programmes than from women who act protectively and stay in treatment programmes.

Despite these limitations, such studies tell us something about the factors influencing women when they discover their child has been sexually abused. The most consistent finding is that women are somewhat less likely to be supportive where the abuser is their current partner than when he is in any other relationship to them (de Jong, 1988; Faller, 1988a; Everson *et al.*, 1989; Sirles and Franke, 1989; Gomes-Schwartz *et al.*, 1990), and also where the abuser is the child's father (de Jong, 1988; Gomes-Schwartz *et al.*, 1990). Only one study appears to have considered the significance of the quality of the mother's own relationship with the child. Women who usually had a caring relationship with their children were most likely to be concerned and protective. Those who had formerly felt hostile to or overburdened by their children were most likely to be angry and unsupportive. A history of dependency on the child to gratify some of their own needs (equally common amongst cases of abuse by father figures and by others) did not appear to affect the mother's response (Gomes-Schwartz *et al.*, 1990). Overall, research has had more success in establishing the influence of current relationships on mothers' responses than in looking to their backgrounds and childhood experiences. The significance of current relationships indicates an important part of the context of women's response. Women's role as mothers involves not only the direct provision of care and protection for dependent children but also the mediation of the conflicting demands and needs of different family members (Graham, 1982). Clearly where child sexual abuse is concerned, the conflicts cannot always be reconciled.

While supportive responses from their mothers aid children's recovery, negative responses, such as anger, disbelief and blame, significantly increase children's distress (Scott and Flowers, 1988; Gomes-Schwartz *et al.*, 1990; Wyatt and Newcomb, 1990; Johnson and Kenkel, 1991). However, it is not only the fact that not all mothers do protect their children which makes women's role as primary protectors in relation to sexual abuse problematic for both women and children. Whatever mothers' responses once they know of sexual abuse by others, their relationship with their children is often damaged by the abuse. Women's role as primary carers and protectors of children underlies this damage as much as it underlies the importance of mothers' support for children. Many children experience feelings of anger and betrayal at their mothers for not having protected them from abuse. Girls who are sexually abused by their fathers are often angrier with their mothers than with the abusers. Such responses are partly the result of children's fantasies that their mothers are all-knowing and all-powerful, derived from their early experience of total dependence on them. To an extent, maternal failure is inevitable against such unrealistic expectations. As Kelly (1988a) has noted, incest survivors are not the only women who feel betrayed by or angry with their mothers. However, such feelings are not necessarily resolved by recognition of the limited powers their mothers have in reality. The anger girls feel may relate as much to the reality of their mothers' relative powerlessness, as to the illusion of their power (Jacobs, 1990).

Sexual abuse confronts children with painful lessons about their own powerlessness, lessons which are often further reinforced for girls by seeing their mothers also dominated by and dependent on men, as well as by the broader context of male dominance. Directing anger towards their mothers serves two purposes. First, anger at their mothers enables girls partially to break their own identification with their mothers, and hence with powerlessness, and to feel worthy of protection from abuse. As such it may play an empowering role in their recovery from abuse, as a temporary stage, prior to the development of a more realistic understanding of their mothers' position and alongside the empowerment of their mothers. Second, however, it is generally easier to direct anger at women than men. As Christine Delphy noted, 'it is precisely the real power of the oppressor . . . which makes him unattackable, or at least not attackable without enormous risks' (1984, p. 121). Since ultimately anger with women is an ineffective response to men's violence, at some point developing a more empowered response involves redirecting anger towards the abuser himself, once it is relatively safe to do so.

The role women play as mothers involves not only protecting children and mediating between family members, but also mediating between family and public agencies (Graham, 1985). As noted above, professionals rely on mothers to prevent children being received into care. Women also seek help from professionals. In Gordon's (1989) historical study of the work of child protection agencies in the USA from 1880–1960 both women and children had frequently initiated intervention. Women sought help in relation to their partners' violence to themselves and their children and when they lacked the resources to care for their own children, although their needs were often reinterpreted by agencies in the intervention process thus set in motion. Today, mothers are one of the main sources of referrals of child sexual abuse to agencies. During the first nine months of the Bexley experiment on joint investigation in child sexual abuse, over half the referrals came from family members, including 28 per cent from mothers and 20 per cent from abused children (Metropolitan Police and Bexley Social Services, 1987). The social control role of state agencies in relation to child protection is often presented as one-way, state against parents (or families) as a unit. In reality it involves two-way negotiations, in which weaker members of the family often seek the help of state agencies to control the abuses of the more powerful.

I have set out this analysis of mothers' roles before discussing the theoretical issues. Much of the mainstream contribution to theoretical debate is based on clinical observation of a small number of cases with severe enough problems not only to have been reported to agencies but also referred to specialists. Much of it is based, too, on the extrapolation of theories derived from therapeutic intervention in child health problems with quite different characteristics. However, it is to the issues raised by these debates that I now turn.

THEORETICAL ISSUES

The role of mothers has been at the centre of conflict between advocates of a family systems (or family dysfunction) approach to child sexual abuse and feminists. There are differences within family systems theory, both theoretical and political, and there is some overlap with feminism now. In a nutshell however, family systems theorists focus on patterns of interaction within families, with a particular emphasis on communication and the psychological roles adopted by family members, and a view of causality as circular, involving all family members. In this model sexual abuse easily becomes seen as an individual response, and hence secondary, to shared problems such as poor communication. Some clinicians now attempt to counter this tendency for the abuse itself to become secondary by combining a family systems perspective with an individual model of sexual abuse as addiction (Furniss, 1991). Nevertheless, family systems theorists have had little if anything to say about the vast majority of incidents of child sexual abuse which occur outside families nor about why it is primarily men rather than women who sexually abuse children. Their analysis is derived from clinical samples and practice, not from research with control groups or community populations. Most versions are based on a functionalist model of the family as a consensual unit in which the sexual division of labour is regarded as natural. There are now theorists however who attempt to combine family systems thinking with feminism, recognising the different experiences of individuals within families, the significance of gender and power in family/household relations, the plurality of family/household forms and the interconnectedness of conflict and inequity within the family/household with structural inequalities in the wider society (Masson and O'Byrne, 1990).

There are also differences and developments within feminism. The common core however is to define child sexual abuse as a social problem, a form of sexual violence sustained (along with rape, sexual harassment and domestic violence) by a male-dominated society in which dominance is eroticised and women and girls are objectified and defined in relation to male needs. Where masculine sexuality is constructed as not requiring reciprocity, the sexual abuse of children is a further extension of non-consensual relationships between peers. The critical period for the development of sexually abusive behaviour appears to be adolescence, and research with community samples has found such behaviour significantly associated with sexist attitudes (Herman, 1988). Moreover, sexually abusive behaviour is not uncommon amongst men – in one study of male college students, one in four acknowledged using some form of coercion to achieve sexual relations with an unwilling partner (Koss *et al.*, 1987). Cross-cultural evidence also suggests that sexually aggressive behaviour in men is significantly related to child rearing arrangements. Where fathers share more equally in the care of children, boys appear to grow up less inclined to aggressive displays of male superiority. Lisak (1991) suggests that it is children's total dependence on women in early childhood which leads later, for boys, to a need to define themselves in opposition to women and that this is reduced by fathers' involvement in child-rearing. However, it may well be boys' expectations (or lack of them) of having a future nurturing role in relation to children themselves which is most significant. There is convincing evidence that male aggression, with distancing from and objectification of women, is fostered in the male peer group, more than in the mother–son relationship (Johnson, 1988).

The main weakness of feminist theory so far has been its failure to address the variability between men. Nevertheless the significance of the broader social context and of adolescence in the development of sexually abusive behaviour indicate that families formed in adulthood are probably not the most important place to look. The role of such families is primarily as the place where offenders most easily get access to children. The attempt to theorise sexual abuse by women from a feminist perspective has also only just begun (Kelly, 1991). The evidence that a small number of women sexually abuse children does not invalidate previous feminist analyses however. Sexual violence remains a predominantly male problem. The importance of feminist theory lies both in taking seriously this current reality and in identifying gender and sexuality as socially constructed and hence variable.

The key issues theoretical debates raise in relation to mothers revolve around whether they are attributed any role in explaining sexual abuse by others, and what responsibility if any they bear for it. It is these questions I consider below, in order both to identify some of the problems in the debate and to set out a framework.

Explanation

Finkelhor (1984) has suggested a model for explaining child sexual abuse (both extrafamilial and intrafamilial) which is now widely accepted by professionals. This sets out four preconditions that have to be met for sexual abuse to occur. A potential abuser needs first to have some motivation to abuse a child sexually, second to overcome internal inhibitions against acting on that motivation, third to overcome external impediments to committing sexual abuse and, fourth, the abuser or some other factor has to undermine or overcome the child's possible resistance to sexual abuse. Explanation requires addressing, first, all four preconditions and, second, the interaction between individual, familial and social factors at each stage. Since offending behaviour can commonly be traced back to adolescence, before the marital relationship was formed, the part mothers may play if this model is adopted is at the third and fourth stage, via the child's supervision and vulnerability. Any contribution women's relationships with their children make to the child's vulnerability is significant only after the abuser is motivated to abuse and has overcome his own internal inhibitions.

MacLeod and Saraga (1991) have questioned this model, arguing that the third and fourth preconditions do not belong within the area of explanation since they are concerned with how and not why offenders abuse. To some extent this is true, but since offenders often target children they perceive to be already vulnerable, the child's prior emotional security and supervision may bear some relation to why that child at that time. A more productive way forward than rejecting altogether the question of why some children are more vulnerable than others would be to locate it in a broader context than the mother–child relationship, as well as recognising that much greater priority should be attached to why offenders abuse. All children are vulnerable to adults to some extent, and no child is supervised all the time. While some children are less supervised and more vulnerable than others, not all of them are sexually abused, and some are sexually abused despite close supervision and close relationships with their mothers.

Some family systems theorists still attribute to mothers a causal role in abuse, although many now stress a distinction between cause and responsibility, arguing that circular causality does not mean that the personal responsibility of the perpetrator for the abuse is lessened or that mothers are to blame for it. Others distinguish between cause and maintenance, suggesting that family dynamics may play a part in maintenance if not cause (Masson and O'Byrne, 1990). Neither of these developments rescue their advocates from the charge that they simply describe family characteristics and interactions, attach technical-sounding labels to them ('syndromes' being particularly popular) and explain nothing. The catch-all concept of circular causality means that all behaviour of family members, however widely it varies, is by definition a part of the problem until the problem is stopped. Within this framework mothers cannot avoid a 'role' in the abuse, whether it is one of not knowing anything about it (and hence the failure of communication between them and the child being the problem) or of suspecting and not taking 'appropriate steps' to stop it (seen as collusion) (Elton, 1988). The substitution of maintenance for cause does not over-come this problem.

The addiction model of child sexual abuse which is now gaining ground in debate offers an alternative way of understanding the other family problems that sometimes accompany sexual abuse, as well as a better base from which to explain abuse itself. If it too errs towards the descriptive, it is at least a more accurate description. Herman's (1988) version of the model offers a way of combining it with feminist social theory. As she points out, sociocultural factors play a major role in creating a climate of risk for addictions of other kinds too. Alcoholism flourishes in cultures that do not allow children to learn safe drinking practices and that glorify or excuse adult drunkenness. Similarly, compulsive sexually abusive be-haviour may be fostered in cultures which do not permit children to learn safely about sex and which glorify or excuse sexual violence. Men also heavily outnumber women in most compulsive anti-social behaviours. The greater social tolerance of anti-social behaviour in men and the im-poverishment in male development of emotional resources may both con-tribute. As Herman puts it:

> Lacking [the emotional resources of intimacy and interdependence], men may be more susceptible to developing dependence on sources of gratification that do not require a mutual relationship with a human being: the bottle, the needle, or the powerless, dehumanized sexual object.
>
> (Herman, 1988, p. 711)

The addiction model offers not only a description of the compulsive quality of some offenders' behaviour but analogies which highlight some of its complexities. The abuse of children, like the use of alcohol, varies from the opportunistic to the highly compulsive and the problem is often not detected until it is well advanced. The concept of addiction captures both the sense of a partial loss of self-control and a continued capacity for exercising it when necessary, for example to avoid detection. Addicts are also well known for their ability to deny their behaviour or rationalise it by blaming others. Such rationalisations – blaming unhappy marriages and childhoods, for example – no longer have credibility in the literature on alcohol abuse where it is recognised that marital dissatisfaction, depression and other situational stresses are commonly the result not the cause of the problem (Herman, 1988). There are important limitations, too, to analogies with drug or alcohol addiction. The exploitation of another person places sexual abuse squarely in the realm of criminal behaviour. Work with offenders also reveals that they commonly plan their access to children in detail (Conte *et al.*, 1989). It may therefore be that the sense they express of compulsiveness is to some extent another form of rationalisation for behaviour from which they derive gratification and which they do not wish to relinquish.

We do not yet have a fully satisfactory explanation of child sexual abuse, which addresses both the interaction between social conditions and individual propensities and the range of offending behaviour. However, the answer to the question I raised earlier of whether mothers of children sexually abused by others should play a part in such an explanation is mostly no. Where it is to any extent yes, it is a minimal one relating only to the vulnerability (but not actual abuse) of a particular child.

Given this analysis of the limited part mothers may play in explaining abuse, it is worth examining one currently popular theory, that there is a 'cycle of abuse' which results in women who have been sexually abused as children themselves being more likely to have children who are sexually abused. This is often presented in enigmatic fashion as if the connection spoke for itself. DiSabatino, for example, comments that 'it is no coincidence that children are often molested around the same age that their mothers were' (1989, p. 17), but declines to specify what mechanism links a woman's childhood experience with her child's experience at the hands of another adult (most probably in her absence).

Cycle of abuse theories are appealing for a number of reasons. First, most professionals probably do come into contact with women whose children have been sexually abused who have also been sexually abused themselves. Given the prevalence of sexual abuse amongst women, it would be surprising if this were not a common experience. The assumption of some causal connection offers a simple focus for work and under-standing, avoiding the complex and emotive issues raised by work with offenders themselves. Such work may well benefit both mother and child, offering an opportunity for the former to resolve past experiences. How-ever, only work with offenders will prevent sexual abuse recurring. Second, they are consistent with professional adherence to a family sys-tems perspective, where reference is sometimes made to sexual abuse being 'repeated across generations' (Vizard and Tranter, 1988, p. 73). Hence professional interests are served by a focus on 'breaking the cycle' in multi-problem families rather than tackling the more intractable but central problem of masculinity. Third, they have an emotional appeal. In most of their forms, cycle of abuse theories transform offenders into victims and hence enable professionals to empathise more easily with them (Herman, 1988). Where mothers of sexually abused children are concerned, however, they serve a different purpose. A non-abusing mother is transformed into a potentially abusing or non-protecting mother by the discovery that she too was abused, making her a legitimate target for change-orientated intervention.

As Herman notes in relation to perpetrators, 'the only serious problem with the "cycle of abuse" concept is its lack of empirical validity' (1988, p. 704). Where mothers of sexually abused children are concerned, such findings as there are which indicate high rates of childhood sexual abuse may to some extent be the result of sample bias. Women often have their own memories of abuse triggered by the discovery of a child's abuse (Courtois and Sprei, 1988; Walker, 1988) and women with a history of abuse themselves may have a greater desire to seek help for their children to spare them effects that they have suffered (Dempster, 1989). Moreover, in all studies reporting a link (Goodwin *et al.*, 1981; Leroi, 1984; Faller, 1989), a substantial proportion, if not the majority, of women whose children have been sexually abused do not report being sexually abused themselves.

Responsibility and power

Much of the debate surrounding women whose children have been sexually abused revolves around blame and responsibility. The overt mother-blaming identified by feminists in the early family dysfunction literature is less common today, but mother-blaming continues in more subtle forms. It is useful to distinguish between two forms. The first – attributing responsibility to women for the sexually abusive behaviour of their partners – could more accurately be called wife-blaming. It is a reworking of the old myth that men are unable to control their sexuality so women must contain it. There can be no justification for this; men deprived of sexual or emotional satisfaction have many other options than to abuse children, and responsibility for the behaviour of adults belongs with the individual adult. Although family systems theorists now commonly stress the personal responsibility of the abuser and deny any intention to blame women, it is likely that their practice still gives subtle (or not so subtle) messages of this kind. Hildebrand, for example, notes that therapeutic work based on a systemic view of causation requires women 'to acknowledge how the marriage relationship or partnership, as well as the structure and organisation of the family, may have contributed to the sexual abuse' (1989, p. 244).

The second form of mother-blaming concerns the degree of responsibility attributed to mothers for the welfare of their children. The problem in this context is not that women are accorded any responsibility but that they are commonly accorded unequal if not sole responsibility. Much apparently gender-neutral discussion of parental responsibilities rests on implicitly gendered assumptions which accord women a disproportionate share. Bentovim *et al.*, for example, have argued that 'a parent who knows that the other parent is in a state of depression, anger or frustration and leaves that parent to care for the child . . . indicates a failure in sharing responsibility' (1987, p. 29). This clearly means mothers leaving depressed fathers. If fathers who left depressed mothers to care for children were cause for state intervention, local authority social services departments (SSDs) would be swamped. More is expected of mothers partly because women are more likely to be socialised to be sensitive to and skilled in dealing with emotional and interpersonal issues. But, as Caplan argues, 'what we should do about that is to take great care to acknowledge what mothers do do, and to expect fathers or other parent figures to do an equal share' (1990, p. 63).

The further problem is that women often lack the resources to exercise their parental responsibilities effectively. Hence, motherhood is characterised by 'powerless responsibility' (Rich, 1977). This is not to say that mothers are wholly without power. The position of women whose children are sexually abused is contradictory in three ways. First, they are frequently both relatively powerless in relation to men, on whom they are often economically dependent, and by whom they are often victimised themselves, and at the same time relatively powerful in relation to their children, whose protection or further abuse is influenced by their actions. While both gender and age are significant axes of power, they are qualitatively different – the power mothers have by virtue of age progressively lessens as their children get older, and in the case of boy children may be counterbalanced by the power children acquire by virtue of their gender. Second, despite the objective power women have in relation to their children, many also express a subjective sense of powerlessness (Hildebrand and Forbes, 1987). Third, their resources (emotional, social and material) are generally depleted by the discovery of the child's abuse and the losses this involves for them, at the same time as the expectations on them are increased by the child's needs and by the demands of professionals.

This last aspect of their position raises the question of what demands are made of women whose children have been sexually abused when they come into contact with state agencies. In considering this, feminists have focused primarily on the pathologising of women in family dysfunction theory. Social work practice however is influenced as much by policy as by theory, although its relationship to neither is direct or self-evident.

THE POLICY CONTEXT

Over the last few years, child sexual abuse has been added in gradually to the policy guidance issued by the Department of Health (DoH) on protecting children from abuse – guidance which is concerned primarily with inter-agency cooperation and with relations between state agencies, parents and children. Local authorities have some discretion in how far they follow this guidance, and some had developed more comprehensive policies on child sexual abuse well in advance of central government. Some local authorities have adopted policies influenced by feminist analysis, and make the distinction between abusing and non-abusing parents (Boushel and Noakes, 1988; Reid, 1989). The DoH, however, has shown only a partial recognition of non-abusing parents and little of feminist analysis. Explicitly, the concept of a non-abusing parent has made two fleeting appearances, first in the guidelines for training Social Services staff on child sexual abuse (DoH, 1989a) and second in the draft version of *Working Together* issued in June 1991 (DoH, 1991a). In both cases, the context involved separation from an offender. Elsewhere parents remained an aggregate unit, equally part of the problem to which professionals relate. The role parents play as protectors was recognised only in relation to child sexual abuse by strangers, where care and support from parents (undivided) might relieve agencies of the need to intervene. There was no recognition of the role one parent may play in protecting children from others within the family and informal networks.

In the final version of *Working Together* (DoH, 1991b), this partial visibility of non-abusing parents has gone. It is replaced however by *implicit* recognition of the existence and role of non-abusing parents in a somewhat wider range of contexts. There is more focus on 'abusers' rather than on parents as a unit, with references alongside to 'other family members' or 'those with parental responsibilities'. There is also increased recognition of potential conflict between parents. However, the shift in approach to abusers is somewhat ambiguous in its implications, and conflict between parents is presented only as an exceptional circumstance. Policy on child sexual abuse is constructed as much by the previous context of child protection work as by these minor adjustments. Hence that context merits brief review.

Child protection policy has been characterised from its nineteenth-century beginnings by the attempt to reconcile contradictory aims – the protection of children from their parents when necessary on the one hand and the reinforcement of family privacy and parental responsibility on the other. The balance struck between these aims has varied at different times, and the most recent legislation, the Children Act 1989, reworks it again, both increasing the grounds for state intervention to protect children and setting out a new framework for partnership with parents geared to the preservation and support of parental responsibilities. The Children Act 1989 followed a series of inquiries during the 1980s which had brought into particularly sharp focus the tightrope professionals concerned with child protection walk in their relations with parents and children. First professionals were accused of focusing too much on the needs of the parents and doing too little too late to protect three children who died at home at the hands of their fathers or stepfathers.[5] Later they were accused of intervening too soon to remove 121 children suspected of being sexually abused in Cleveland from their parents, and overlooking the need to work with parents for the sake of the children.[6] The policy recommendations of these inquiries, along with policy guidance issued by the DoH and the new legislation, refer throughout to gender-neutral parents. There is no recognition of either the role mothers may play in protecting children from both physical and sexual abuse by fathers or stepfathers or the difficulties they face in doing so when they are often victimised by and dependent on these men themselves.[7] Acceptance of the sexual division of labour as natural and unproblematic means women are expected to protect their children from violent men with little help from state agencies and risk losing their children when they fail.

During the 1980s professionals were urged both to use greater authority against parents and to work in partnership with them. The DoH (1988) attempted to reconcile these aims with a model of practice it referred to as 'therapeutic control'. It argued that past concerns about the tensions between care and control in the social work role were misguided, for 'it is now generally agreed that care and control, as any parent knows, are part of the same process' (1988, p. 11). In this model of the state as parent and the family as a rather difficult child, parents are again presented as a unit. Neither the different interests of individuals within the family and the consequent two-way negotiations over social control that occur between family members and agencies, nor the historical trend towards a greater use of compulsion with parents since the mid-1970s are acknowledged. The latter trend predated the Thatcher government and was initially a response to the death in 1973 of Maria Colwell.[8] However, it was exacerbated by broader economic changes and the restructuring of the state's role in welfare from 1979.

The model of practice now advocated by the DoH places increased emphasis on social work assessments as a way of separating the truly 'dangerous' or 'high risk' parents, with whom intervention is necessary to protect children, from the rest who can be left to themselves. Services are intended to be more treatment-orientated, by implication only for parents with particular problems, with the law providing a necessary framework. This model is based on one developed by the Rochdale team of the NSPCC (Dale *et al.*, 1986), in which intervention is clearly intended to be short term. Parents are given a relatively short time to prove themselves to experts, with a return to parental independence the goal. It is both a more residual model and one more pessimistic about the possibilities of change than the preventive orientation of the 1960s. It also assumes a knowledge base – to predict accurately the 'high risk' – which does not exist in a form adequate to the task.

The 'therapeutic control' model of practice may well have had limited influence in many local authorities. However, where SSDs wish to continue to offer longer-term and preventive services, their capacity to do so has gradually been curtailed through the 1980s by resource shortages. In London, there were 600 children on child protection registers without an allocated social worker in 1988, rising to 820 in 1989 – about 10 per cent of the total (Second Report of the Commons Health Committee, 1991). In this context, the social work role is increasingly one of surveillance only, and assessment becomes primarily a way of prioritising demands on limited resources. Since child care is regarded as primarily women's responsibility, it is on women that such policing falls. It is also women's capacities in providing care which are the main focus of assessment. The implications of this trend are therefore towards both greater surveillance and greater expectations of women.

It is in this context that the changes in policy in response to child sexual abuse must be considered. Two changes of particular significance to women whose children have been sexually abused have occurred, both of which have been advocated by feminists in the interests of both women and children. First, it has been recommended that, where possible, suspected offenders should be removed from the home rather than abused children. Second, the concept of a non-abusing parent has received some (if transient) official recognition. In the current context and in the form they have taken however, these are a somewhat mixed blessing. In the draft version of *Working Together* (DoH, 1991a), the onus for the removal of offenders was placed primarily on women, who could apply for a court order under domestic violence legislation. The experience of women attempting to escape partners violent to themselves indicates that in practice this legislation does not currently provide effective protection. One recent study found that only about half the women who applied for civil protection through the courts achieved what they asked for. Of those who did achieve an order or 'undertaking', again only about half found it effective in preventing further violence or harassment from their partners (Barron, 1990). The draft guidelines also referred to provision made in the Children

Act 1989 for local authorities to provide accommodation for an alleged abuser who leaves the home.

In the final version of *Working Together* (DoH, 1991b), three changes were made relevant to the issue of removal. First, the onus for achieving it was shifted from women to the police. While this indicates that state agencies are to take a greater share of responsibility, where the police decide not to make an arrest some women will continue to rely on domestic violence legislation. No attention has been given to improving its effectiveness. Second, it is argued that removal alone is too simplistic a solution to a complex problem. This is undoubtedly so, but moving on to the politically easier ground of professional work with abusers leaves the continuing problems surrounding removal itself unaddressed. Third, the reference to local authorities providing accommodation for an alleged abuser who leaves the home has been dropped. In practice, the exclusion of abusers from further access to the child is likely to continue to depend primarily on the mother's determination to prevent it.

The existence of non-abusing parents was explicitly recognised by the DoH only within the context of separation from an offender (DoH, 1989a, 1991a). An increased focus on abusers entails an implicit move away from seeing parents as an aggregate unit elsewhere. However, the position of a non-abusing mother is made less visible by the language of 'other family members' or 'those with parental responsibilities' (who include, of course, abusing parents). While there is now some recognition of conflict between parents, specifically in the context of parental attendance at case conferences, this nettle has been grasped very tentatively. Conflict is presented solely at the level of the individual couple, with no acknowledgement of its context in structural inequalities or of women's relative powerlessness both within families and within society. The guidance clearly aims to minimise the implications of disaggregating parents.

Women have increasingly been encouraged to separate from abusing partners to prevent sexually abused children being received into care. At the same time, rising case loads and scarce resources in SSDs mean that mothers who do separate from an abusing partner are likely to be low priority for further help. Since separation usually involves financial losses for women, recognition of non-abusing parents in this context is likely, for many women, to mean that their responsibilities increase while their resources are depleted. This is far short of an approach to child protection policy which would empower women to support their children and aim to enable rather than simply assess. A more positive trend has been the increasing recognition amongst professionals that building alliances with women whose children have been sexually abused is vital to successful intervention, and that such alliances demand attention to the needs of mothers as well as of children. A number of local initiatives – primarily self-help groups – have been reported in the social work press.[9] However, where local authorities have developed more comprehensive policies – for example, to allocate a social worker each to both mother and child – their ability to implement them is constrained by the resource context.

It is not only child protection policy which influences women's ability to protect their children. Both the criminal law and civil court actions after divorce are also important. Very few cases of child sexual abuse currently result in prosecution, despite recent changes in the rules of evidence and in legal procedure to facilitate this.[10] It is commonly assumed that women do not want abusive partners prosecuted and that it is fear of this outcome which inhibits them from reporting abuse to the police. Women's hopes and expectations of the legal system are more complex and variable than this however, as Chapters 6 and 7 show. In practice, the failure of the state to take effective action against abusers increases women's responsibilities for protecting children from men's violence.

Women who divorce abusive partners might be thought to have achieved effective protection. However, abusive men may apply to the courts for an order to increase their access to children, and ironically it may be becoming more difficult for women to protect children in these cir-cumstances. The Children Act 1989 has changed the framework and the language within which parents' relationships with children after divorce are adjudicated. Custody and access orders have been replaced by the concept of parental responsibility, which both parents retain after divorce, and specific orders on residence and contact. The problem however remains the same. A new myth has developed that women make false and malicious allegations of sexual abuse against their ex-partners in the con-text of custody and access disputes.[11] This myth makes little sense. Child sexual abuse is far too difficult to prove to provide an easy way of winning such a dispute. It is also not supported by research. The incidence of sexual abuse reported in families involved in contested custody and access cases does appear to be slightly higher than in the general population. However this could be expected for a number of reasons. First, the discovery of child sexual abuse often results in separation or divorce. Second, children are more vulnerable to sexual abuse in the context of separation or divorce, both by their fathers and other men. Third, children are more able to tell of past abuse when an abusive father has left, because of their own greater safety and their mother's decreased dependence on and trust in him. The most comprehensive piece of research so far on allegations of sexual abuse in the context of custody and access disputes has found no evidence that they are more likely to be found false in this than in any other context (Thoennes and Tjaden, 1990). Many allegations remain unsubstantiated, but this is not the same as being false.[12] The myth however demonstrates that mothers face a similar dilemma to social workers – they have been blamed in the past for not taking action, and now they risk being blamed if they do.

OUTLINE OF THE BOOK

Earlier in this chapter, the findings of the small but growing body of research on women's responses to the sexual abuse of their children were outlined. Most of these studies have attempted to establish factors predictive of different types of response. They have had some, but not great, success in doing so. Their relevance to professionals is limited. The discovery of certain factors with some predictive power offers little to the task of influencing response. Building alliances between workers and mothers to enable mothers to support their children where possible requires a better understanding of the processes involved in women's responses. It also requires an understanding developed 'from the inside'. Unless workers can understand mothers' own definitions of their situation, no dialogue is likely to be established from which to work, if necessary, towards change.

The study on which this book is based was a qualitative one, focusing not on predicting outcomes but on exploring processes. The losses involved for women in the sexual abuse of a child are described first (in Chapter 3), since loss was an ongoing theme influencing the processes of finding out about abuse (Chapter 4), of deciding what to do (Chapter 5) and of seeking help (Chapter 6). Some of the women interviewed had moved quickly through these processes, some had moved more slowly and some had not moved very far at all. The aim of the study was to explore the nature of the processes in depth, identify what factors appeared to contribute to movement, and locate all responses in the context of their meaning in each woman's life. Each chapter ends with a summary identifying issues relating to the interpretation of women's responses, similarities with the processes engaged in by child protection workers and the implications of this analysis for ways of influencing women's responses. Chapters 6 and 7 then discuss the women's experiences of the responses of others, both informal and formal sources of help. First, however, the aims and methodology of the study are elaborated.

2 The study
Aims and methods

My study was designed to explore the processes involved for women in finding out about the sexual abuse of their children, deciding what to do about the family relationships involved (both short and long term) and about involving others, and their experience of others' responses, from both informal sources and professional agencies. The focus both on processes that developed over time and on the women's own interpretations of their experience indicated that depth interviewing was the most appropriate method. As Jones suggests:

> In order to understand why persons act as they do we need to understand the meaning and significance they give to their actions. The depth interview is one way of doing so. . . . For to understand other persons' constructions of reality we would do well to ask them (rather than assume we can know merely by observing their overt behaviour) and to ask them in such a way that they can tell us in their terms.
>
> (Jones, 1985b, p. 46)

The main source of data on which this study draws is therefore a sample of interviews, tape-recorded and transcribed in full, with fifteen women whose children had been sexually abused.

I initially defined the sample as including women whose children had been sexually abused by a trusted adult, within or outside the family. At the time the study was set up, the existing research on mothers' responses focused on abuse by fathers or stepfathers only (Myer, 1984; Johnson, 1985). It seemed likely that there would be some similar issues with abuse by other relatives and possibly by others. Later research has confirmed that this is so (de Jong, 1988; Sirles and Franke, 1989; Regehr, 1990), but in fact all the women who volunteered to be interviewed had children who had been sexually abused by members of the household or non-resident kin (not all of whom were adults). The cases therefore all fall within Faller's

(1988b) definition of intrafamilial abuse. The distinctiveness of this category is worth retaining. Where the category of incest (implying blood relationship) is replaced by 'abuse in the home' to emphasise the greater significance of access (La Fontaine, 1990), there is a danger of losing sight of the long-term issues of access that may be involved with all kin, whether resident or not.

I also initially planned to interview thirty women, but reduced the number to fifteen, partly because of the difficulty of collecting a sample at all, and partly because the interviews were often extremely long (up to five hours) and took up to three days each to transcribe. The nature of the subject raised particular problems for contacting a sample. Retrospective surveys of adults indicate that the vast majority of incidents of child sexual abuse go unreported to agencies of any kind. There was no obvious point of contact for unreported cases. Furthermore, where records existed of reported cases (such as those of SSDs) there were problems of how to make contact without intrusion. It would for instance have been totally inappropriate to obtain names from agencies and write to women direct, indicating that their expectations of confidentiality with the agency concerned had already been breached.

Both the sensitivity of the subject and the aim of depth interviewing meant it was important that women participated voluntarily. I also hoped to interview women who had been in contact with agencies and those who had not, and to include middle-class and working-class women. American research indicates no significant social class or black–white differences in the prevalence of sexual abuse, although reported cases are overwhelmingly biassed towards working-class families (Finkelhor, 1986a). I was not aiming for a sample representative of all mothers of sexually abused children in contact with agencies (which would have replicated this bias) or of all women whose children had been sexually abused (which would have demanded a screening exercise beyond my resources), but to explore a range of experiences. I therefore used a variety of methods for collecting the sample, negotiating access via SSDs and voluntary organisations, and placing letters in women's magazines. A similar approach to collecting a sample has been used in other exploratory studies of sensitive subjects. A letter in *Everywoman* magazine produced two women who were willing to participate. Contact with three voluntary organisations who agreed to pass a letter from me on to women they knew produced another four. Six SSDs also agreed to participate, and the remainder were contacted via them. Both voluntary and statutory agencies were asked to explain to the women concerned that they had given me no information themselves and it was for them to choose to contact me if they were willing to participate in the research. A minimum time lapse of six months from their discovery of abuse before they were approached was set to avoid intrusion on the early stages of loss and confusion they were likely to be experiencing.

Each woman was offered a preliminary interview, which would not be tape-recorded, in which I would explain more fully the aims of the research and what participation would involve and they could ask questions. They could then decide after meeting me whether to participate. At the same time, I sent all women who replied to my letter details of counselling services they might contact for help if they wished, whether or not they participated, in an attempt to avoid any confusion between research and counselling. In practice, every woman who agreed to meet had already decided to talk, and it was sometimes difficult for me to say anything before they started.

Women who participated did so for three main reasons. The most common was to help others, to put their experience to use in some way. Very nearly as common, though less often stated explicitly, was the need for recognition of their own experience, to be heard, recorded and believed. This was revealed in a number of ways. One woman remarked when I outlined the aims of the research that no one would be interested, 'no one cares about the mother, no one seems to have thought what it's like for the mother'. Another referred to the transcript of her interview as her 'statement' and went through it in great detail to ensure it was correct as if it might prove some sort of protection against the disbelief of others. A third reason for participating was simply for someone to talk to. Most of the women had not talked about their experience in such depth before, and the offer of a neutral listener was therefore welcome. The sense of being listened to however was rare enough for most to be disturbing as well as a relief – several of the interviews included long pauses for tears or silence, as distressing memories emerged.

THE SAMPLE

The method of contacting respondents meant that the fifteen women interviewed comprise a collection of cases which is not representative either of the general population of women with children or of mothers of sexually abused children. The characteristics of the sample and details of the forms of abuse involved are outlined here. In the following chapters, the women are identified by initials when their case is discussed at length or quoted, and brief case summaries given in the Appendix allow reference to key variables to be made.

Thirteen of the fifteen women had been married at least once, the two others having had long-term cohabiting relationships which they had hoped would lead to marriage but which had ended before the interviews. Eight were currently married or cohabiting at the time of the interviews (three to first husbands, four to second husbands or cohabitees and one to a fourth). Seven were currently living without a partner. Of these, six had had a single long-term relationship or marriage and one had had two. Overall then, nine of the women had had only one marriage-type relationship. Two were in their twenties, nine in their thirties, one in her forties and three in their fifties. The time elapsed from their discovery of the child's abuse to the interview varied from slightly less than six months to thirteen years. Their discoveries therefore spanned the period from 1974 to 1987.

Assessing women's social class position is not straightforward.[1] Eleven of the women in this sample have been grouped as working class. Of these however, the categorisation was unambiguous for seven, who had come from working-class backgrounds, done manual occupations themselves and married or lived with men in working-class occupations. Of the other four, three had done non-manual clerical work themselves at some time either before or during the marriage but came from working-class families and were married to men in manual occupations. The fourth had married her husband at a time when he had been promoted to non-manual work (from which he was made redundant later), but both she and her husband came from working-class backgrounds and her own occupations had been predominantly manual. Four of the women have been categorised broadly as middle class. For two this was unambiguous since they came from middle-class families, had done middle-class jobs prior to marriage and married men in middle-class occupations. For two however, one of these three factors was working class – one coming from a working-class family of origin and the other having married a man with a manual occupation. In both cases their orientation seemed predominantly middle class.

Two of the working-class women were Afro-Caribbean in origin, both having come to Britain as children. The other thirteen women were white, of British origin. The sample is not large enough to identify the significance of differences of either class or race systematically in the analysis. Where there seemed possible links, these have been indicated – for example, in the influence of money on decisions to separate (see Chapter 5). For most of the analysis however the women are discussed as a whole group. This is not to imply that women's experience is not significantly differentiated by race and class, but the exploration of the significance of such differences to women's responses to the sexual abuse of a child was beyond the scope of this study.

In eleven of the fifteen cases, the abuser was the woman's partner (husband, ex-husband or cohabitee) and in four, other relatives (one the woman's father, one her son, and two relatives of her partner – uncles or cousins to the child). Fourteen of the children were girls and one a boy. Nine of the children had been aged five or under at the time the abuse started, two between six and ten, and four aged eleven to thirteen. In thirteen cases the abuse was continuous, for periods ranging from under six months to over ten years. In four of the families it was possible but not certain that siblings had also been abused as well as the child known to have been sexually abused.

Of the eleven women whose partners or ex-partners had been the abuser, two were still living with them, two had separated before they discovered the abuse and seven separated after discovering the abuse. Of the latter seven, only three separated almost immediately the abuse was discovered however and, of these three, one had already been through four years of suspicions before that point. The process involved in decisions to separate is discussed further in Chapter 5. Two of the children were permanently in care, and a third temporarily in care, due to return home shortly at the time of the first interview. At the last contact she had returned home, but her future was still uncertain. Nine of the children were still living with their mother (including all the four abused by relatives other than the woman's partner), one, by then aged 26, was still living with her father (the abuser), and two had left home because of age. In one of these last two cases, the parents were still together and the daughter still visited.

The tables below give further details of the forms the abuse took, the circumstances in which it occurred and the legal response.

Table 1 refers to a total of fifteen children, twelve of whom were subjected to two or more forms of sexual abuse. This records the types of

Table 1 Types of abuse

Vaginal rape	6
Handling child's genitals	6
Exposure of abuser's genitals to child	5
Masturbation over child's body	5
Oral rape (fellatio)	4
Digital penetration of vagina/anus	2
Other touching of child's body	2
Oral contact with child's genitals	1
Anal rape (buggery)	1
Masturbation of adult by child	1
Showing child pornography	1

abuse known – in several cases, the women did not know the full details of what had happened. The cases included a range of forms of abuse, in a variety of combinations. The two most common forms of abuse were vaginal rape and handling the child's genitals.

It has recently been suggested that the term child sexual abuse covers too many different activities to be useful and that it should be replaced by reference to the specific sexual activities involved (O'Hagan, 1989). There are however both practical and theoretical reasons for continuing to use the broad term child sexual abuse. Given that abuse by family members often continues over a period of months or years and involves a number of different forms, and further that there is nearly always some degree of uncertainty amongst professionals about the full extent of abuse involved, it is both impractical and potentially misleading to refer to the particular form of abuse. Conceptually, while greater specificity may be valuable, it is equally important to recognise the similarities in the experience of different forms of abuse. Finkelhor and Browne (1988) suggest that the initial and long-term effects illustrate traumagenic dynamics common to the many different acts: traumatic sexualisation, stigmatisation, betrayal and powerlessness. An alternative, but not incompatible, model focuses on conditioned anxiety and socially learned responses to the victimisation experience (Berliner and Wheeler, 1987). Furthermore, too much emphasis should not be placed on the sexual act, given the evidence that the relationship and access of the perpetrator to the child and the degree of aggression involved may be equally if not more significant in the harm the child suffers (Wyatt and Powell, 1988; Gomes-Schwartz *et al.*, 1990).

Table 2 Circumstances of abuse

Child's home, mother out (abuser responsible for child)	7
Child's home, mother in	3
Child's home, mother sometimes in, sometimes out	3
Abuser's home, not child's (child visiting relative)	2

In the majority of cases, the woman was not in the same house when the abuse of the child occurred. Of the three cases in which abuse occurred regularly while the mother was in the house, two of the women had been in a different room at the time of the abuse, and the third had been in bed asleep when her husband abused the child in the same bed.

Two of the children had been abused by two perpetrators, and there were therefore seventeen men and boys involved. Of these, only four were

Table 3 Legal action taken

Prosecution and conviction	4
Police involved: no prosecution	9
No police involvement	4

prosecuted, all successfully. Of these four, two pleaded guilty and received a probation order and one month prison sentence respectively. The other two received prison sentences of four years (after pleading guilty to minor charges in exchange for dropping major ones) and seven years respectively.

INTERVIEWING

An interviewing guide was constructed drawing on the literature and on informal discussions with professionals and voluntary organisations who provided counselling for women whose children had been sexually abused. Two pilot interviews revealed the difficulty of imposing a semi-structured format, and an unstructured, story-telling approach was adopted thereafter. This meant starting each interview with one standard question, 'Is there an obvious place for you to start in thinking about what happened to your child?', and following the woman's lead from there. Some of the women started with their own discovery of the abuse, others with the start of their relationship with the abuser, and one with her own experience of abuse in childhood. In some interviews I asked very few questions other than to prompt.

Story telling as a method of interviewing gives more control over the process to the interviewee and also allows experience to be related in context, instead of fractured by the interviewer's questions (Cornwell, 1984; Graham, 1984). The way women chose to tell their stories indicated a great deal about the meaning of their experience to them and their way of coping with it. This method also allowed them to approach painful subjects at their own pace, and to veer away from them as necessary. Graham suggests that opportunities offered for avoiding the truth in story telling can be seen positively as providing space for those who receive researchers into personal areas of their lives. As she points out:

> The switch from the personal testimony to the extravagant tale is not difficult to detect, yet it provides the teller with a way of controlling the release of information about herself. In a situation of inequality, both honest stories and fabricated tales are resources by which informants can redress the balance of power.
>
> (Graham, 1984, p. 120)

Interviewees did certainly use the story-telling mode to maintain control, to the extent of one interviewee several times refusing my questions, saying 'I'll come to that in a minute' or 'That comes later'. While I only occasionally felt fabrication was used, more commonly patches where memory failed indicated those issues which were still particularly painful. I did not pursue questioning when such lapses occurred although often the woman herself came back to such questions at a later point.

Depth interviewing requires the establishment of trust in the interviewer. In order to give, as far as possible, honest accounts of their personal lives, people need to believe in the research and the researcher's commitment to and interest in them (Jones, 1985a). This inevitably means adapting the style of interviewing to the particular individual, knowing when to ask questions and when to listen, checking meaning as appropriate, finding a balance between following and directing the story, and sensing what areas are off limits. I used the original interview schedule to remind me of the areas I hoped to cover. Although I often did not use the specific questions in the schedule, with all interviewees each area was covered. I also always answered questions of information where I had or could obtain the answers.

I planned to interview each woman twice, to tape-record all interviews and to return transcripts of the first interview to them before meeting for the second time (about a month later). Two interviews seemed necessary for several reasons. First, the length of the interview schedule with which I started and the aim of collecting life histories was likely to make a single interview very long. The first pilot interview took five hours and I was anxious to avoid repeating this too often. In the event, it was difficult to restrict the length of the first interviews, given the need to tell the story from beginning to end for women who had in most cases never spoken about their experience in depth before. The shortest was two and a half hours, and on average the first interviews lasted three and a half hours, with five lasting four hours or more. Second, the story-telling mode meant that the order varied considerably in different interviews and a second interview allowed me to check through the transcript for areas that had not been covered or issues I wished to clarify and to raise these on meeting again.

Third, I had hoped that returning transcripts of their first interview to women might increase a sense of participation and allow them some benefit from the process, and in addition serve as a trigger to memory, resulting in further information in the second interview.[2] While it did serve the second purpose, the first was more problematic. Some women valued having the transcript primarily as a weapon in the battle for validation of their experience with others. These women had either shown it to someone else or anticipated doing so, and felt it would provide proof that someone had believed them and taken them seriously. Inevitably, its performance did not always live up to this promise. Some also treated checking the transcript as an extra obligation, despite reporting that reading it had been distressing, raising again painful memories they preferred to forget. As I became aware of these problems, I stressed that there was no obligation to read the transcripts but continued to offer them. All except one of the women interviewed wanted a copy, but five had read only parts of it by the time we met for the second interview.

Fourth, second interviews were important in establishing trust. Given the emotional intensity of the first interviews, and the sense of guilt and shame attached to some of the experiences women were recounting, ending them with discussion of when to meet again demonstrated a commitment to the women and to understanding their experience and helped to normalise the interaction before leaving. In several cases, the second interviews were more relaxed and the trust that had built up allowed different issues to emerge and further questions to be asked.

Finally, second interviews allowed some assessment of how issues were changing. In some cases accounts changed because of changes in the interviewing relationship, where issues emerged that had clearly been there at the time of the first interviews. In others, changes had occurred since the first interview, and it was therefore possible to explore the process by which perceptions of the woman's relationship with the abuser or explanations of the abuse, for instance, changed as she came to terms with it.

In practice it was not possible to interview every woman a second time. Twelve of the women were interviewed twice and the second interviews were generally somewhat shorter than the first, although they still averaged over two hours each and the longest was four hours. Three women were unavailable for a second interview. In one case the woman said she would not meet a second time at the end of the first interview, expressing an impatience with continued talking. She had also had difficulty in participating at all since her husband was violent and possessive and objected to her giving her address to anyone. He was in prison at the time of the first interview but due out shortly. It might well have endangered her to pursue her further. In the other two cases the women initially agreed to meet a second time. One then replied three times to letters attempting to arrange a time, each time saying that she would prefer to defer meeting until her life was more settled but letting me know how she and her daughter were. The second made two further arrangements for follow-up interviews at her home but went out on both occasions. I wrote to her a third time but received no reply.

ANALYSIS

Analysis of qualitative data is always a personal activity involving interpretation as well as the attempt to understand and represent faithfully the world of research participants as they construct it (Jones, 1985b). The themes of the chapters which follow were identified by a case study method – identifying the key processes in one account and then searching others for similar or dissimilar processes and themes (Mitchell, 1983). The transcripts of interviews were then read and each account summarised separately for each chapter, in relation to the theme of that chapter, noting reference to passages which illustrated particular aspects. These summaries enabled the retention of context as expressed by the whole accounts for the analysis of each chapter. Categories were then drawn from the summaries and coded separately again and those which were amenable to quantitative analysis were coded onto spreadsheets. Each transcript was read altogether at least four times. In addition I transcribed all interviews myself and had therefore listened to the tapes repeatedly to do so.

Extracting the essence from pages of uninterrupted text, often with minute details of interactions and dialogue, and with little relation to the chronology of events was a time-consuming task. Not only did the accounts range backwards and forwards in time, in some of them the sense of chronology itself was obscure owing to the unresolved sense of loss involved. While on one level it was possible to reconstruct the accounts in chronological order, on another it was also necessary to consider the meaning of time itself as expressed in the construction of the accounts.

All accounts serve a purpose, actively constructing a version of reality (Potter and Wetherell, 1987). The analysis involved consideration of the relationship of these versions to their contexts, in the woman's life, the interview situation and the broader social context. Individual life histories are rarely simply the recording of events, but involve the interpretation of the past to make sense of the present. They therefore vary as the present changes, and accounts need to be understood in terms of their current meaning in a person's biography. The interview itself, in which the researcher is often seen as an expert to whom a 'best face' should be shown, may also influence accounts, and the broader social context influences what is thought to be a 'best face'. For example, women frequently made remarks such as 'I can't understand mothers who don't believe their children', 'It's natural to protect your children' or 'You have to put your children first' when other parts of their account indicated that their experience had not been anything like as simple as this implied. Such remarks are indicative of the dominant discourse of motherhood. At the same time, they indicate the degree to which the women felt threatened in their identity as mothers and their need to reassert themselves as good mothers, as distinct from other 'bad mothers'.

Both the women's prior contact with agencies and the high level of media coverage during the period of the interviewing were influences on their accounts. Several times, on checking what women meant by a particular version of events – 'She doesn't trust me because I failed to protect her' or 'I was my mother's scapegoat', for instance – I received the reply 'Well, that's what I've been told'. Interpretations of a 'best face' varied, reflecting the conflicting constructions of motherhood present in public debate as well as professional practice. In some accounts there was a somewhat ritualistic expression of guilt, 'I'm to blame because I'm her mother', reflective of the professional discourse of child protection. One woman, however, who had been in contact with a feminist support group, seemed to consider an image of total innocence, victim status and disillusion with all men as the appropriate 'best face', despite her obvious pride in the new husband she had acquired since parting from the abuser six months previously.

My own and other people's reactions to the subject also influenced my analysis. I had worked for five years in a rape crisis centre before starting the research and was already aware of the extent and nature of sexual violence. Nevertheless I came to realise that the emotional impact of exposure to child sexual abuse is intense and far-reaching, and not easily exhausted. My need to retain some distance from the subject made it difficult to transcribe the tapes or re-read the transcripts on occasions. People to whom I talked of the research also often found the subject anxiety-provoking and had a variety of ways of distancing, including avoidance and blame. This made me aware that women whose children are sexually abused have few of the options to distance that the rest of us are able to employ.

3 Loss
The meaning of child sexual abuse to mothers

There are two key findings from previous research on mothers' responses to the sexual abuse of their children. First, there is evidence that they experience trauma themselves, and their reactions and responses have been likened to the process of bereavement (Myer, 1984), the aftermath of rape (de Jong, 1988) or of child sexual abuse itself (Dempster, 1989; Hubbard, 1989). Since women's own experience of sexual violence has been conceptualised as one of loss (Hopkins and Thompson, 1984; Kelly, 1988a), these are not incompatible findings. Second, there are studies which show that the support of mothers is a highly significant factor – if not the most significant factor – affecting the child's healing (Wyatt and Mickey, 1987; Conte and Berliner, 1988; Everson *et al.*, 1989) and that the absence of support from the mother has significantly detrimental effects (Scott and Flowers, 1988).

This combination, of their own trauma and the significance of their support for another's well-being, is not unique to women whose children are sexually abused. It has been suggested that every child or adult who is raped or sexually abused may have on average three significant others who are affected with grief-type responses and who commonly include the main sources of support of the person victimised. These can be seen as secondarily victimised and their recovery does not necessarily match with that of the person primarily victimised (Remer and Elliott, 1988b). This chapter explores, first, the nature of the experience of secondary victimisation as it affects women whose children are sexually abused and, second, the relevance of their own experiences of primary victimisation.

Some of the responses women described are similar to those noted in others who are secondarily victimised. Men whose wives are raped, for instance, may internalise the rape as a threat to their self-image and sense of masculinity, and relationships are vulnerable to breakdown from the mismatch between the recovery processes of those primarily and secondarily victimised (Remer and Elliott, 1988b). The position of mothers is however different from that of many others secondarily victimised in four main ways. First, the losses involved are more extensive, especially where their partners are the abusers. Many others secondarily victimised have no relationship at all with the perpetrator of abuse. Mothers often have a long history of their own relationship with the perpetrator (longer in many cases than that with the child and often to some extent the reason for having had the child). Second, women's psychological development means that, more than for men, loss of attachments are experienced as a loss of self (Baker Miller, 1988). Together with the identification of women with family, this means that the disruption of family relationships which the discovery of sexual abuse triggers may be intensely threatening. Third, the expectation that a good mother should be able to prevent harm to her child means women commonly feel (and are regarded as) implicated in the occurrence of the abuse. And, fourth, their position is different from that of many others secondarily victimised in the extent of support expected from them in the aftermath for the child primarily victimised. The expectations of motherhood are defined by ever-changing child needs (Graham, 1982). Women whose children are sexually abused by a partner are expected to choose between child and partner – a choice which they have often not anticipated ever having to make, and one which is actively discouraged by the social organisation of child rearing with its dominant assumption that women will combine child-care responsibilities (unpaid) with economic dependence on men.

The accounts of the women interviewed for this study indicated that the concept of secondary victimisation – focusing on their ongoing relationships with the victimised children – was necessary but not sufficient to represent the meaning of their experience. Their own experiences of victimisation were also an important part of the context in which the meaning of the child's abuse for them was constructed. In focusing on victimisation, it is not intended to attach to mothers a whole identity or status as victim. Victimisation is a process which women can and do resist (Kelly, 1988a). It is also a process which inhibits their ability to protect their children.

The overarching theme of this chapter is the experience of loss. The sources of loss were multiple and ongoing, and there was a strong sense of endlessness in the women's accounts of their experience, summed up in the phrase of one woman who started her account, 'There's not really a beginning, and there's no end' (RD). Women's experience when a child is sexually abused is best conceptualised as a series of losses extending over time through the life course. The women interviewed described losses of trust in the man who abused the child and more broadly in a just world, of control over their own and their child's life, of ideas of family unity and togetherness and of the past and the future, of their identity as good mothers and, where the abuser was their partner and had seemed to favour the child over themselves, of their sense of femininity. There were losses too of a sense of normality, of home and family as places of safety, and of privacy when others became involved. Overall there was a strong sense that a whole world view was threatened, that the assumptions of shared understandings, trust and the predictability of behaviour on which everyday life and interaction depend, had been overturned. Within this, the meaning of women's experience was constructed within the context of the particular relationships involved and therefore varied.

Losses which disrupt the pattern of attachments within which people construct the meaning of their lives disrupt the ability to experience life as meaningful and induce grief, however rational the changes may seem from the point of view of someone with other attachments (Marris, 1986). The recovery from grief involves reconstituting meaning by rebuilding the continuity of life, making sense of what has happened and assimilating it to present circumstances in a purposeful way. Myer (1984) suggests that 'pathological' outcomes result when women become 'stuck' in one of the stages of bereavement and, for instance, never overcome denial. My study suggested however that 'stuckness' was not adequately represented by a single emotional state but may involve a combination of denial, anger, guilt and depression. Marris's conceptualisation of grieving as a process involving the need to reconcile conflicting impulses (to return to the time before the loss occurred and to reach forward to a state of mind where the loss is forgotten) was more useful. Where grief is unresolved, the conflicting claims of past and future are unreconciled (Marris, 1986). Adopting this analysis of grief, 'stuckness' in these women's accounts was judged on the basis of clinging to the pre-abuse (or pre-marriage) past (often idealised) and/or the possibility of future revenge/vindication ('biding my time') accompanied by little or no meaning attached to the present. In contrast, women who had more or less resolved their losses ranged in their accounts more easily between past, present and future, but constructed the meaning of their lives primarily from the present. This is not an all-or-nothing distinction but one of degree. Not only is grieving a process, but the losses are ongoing and those women who felt they had more or less accepted the abuse, still felt it would 'always be there'. Moreover, since there are multiple sources of loss, some women had resolved some but not others.

The need to re-establish continuity of self was amply demonstrated by the way women told their stories. Despite my initial anxiety that asking questions about many aspects of their own lives might imply blame, given the space to construct their own stories, these women ranged over their whole lives including their childhood attachments in their families of origin, and past, current and anticipated future relationships with husbands and partners, children and close friends, within which meaning was primarily constructed for them. While the need to reconstruct meaning and continuity is useful as an overarching framework for coming to terms with loss, Breakwell's typology of coping strategies adopted in response to threatened identity informed the analysis of women's responses to specific situations. Coping strategies are defined by their goal, as ways of preventing, avoiding or controlling distress. They may involve a variety of responses which change the situation that causes distress, change the meaning of the situation or control the stress once it has occurred: 'Any thought or action which succeeds in eliminating or ameliorating threat can be considered a coping strategy whether it is consciously recognised as intentional or not' (Breakwell, 1986, p. 79). The third section of this chapter considers the implications of a model focusing on their own losses for understanding women's responses to the sexual abuse of their children.

SECONDARY VICTIMISATION

The process of secondary victimisation revolves centrally around an on-going relationship with the person primarily victimised. Both the actual and anticipated effects of sexual abuse on the child (as well as the broader disruption of family relationships involved) meant there were long-term implications for mothers. Most made comments indicating a sense that sexual abuse, unlike other forms of child injury, was an irrevocable event, which would affect the child (and consequently themselves) for life. 'It will never ever go away. It's not like when they fall over and break their leg, you help the leg to repair and then you forget more or less. This is something different' (AN). Those women who felt their children were on some level 'over it' and not showing obvious effects of the abuse were more able to regain control of their lives, but still felt it would 'always be there'. There are similarities with the accounts of others secondarily victimised in relation to rape and sexual abuse – the adjustment process is painful, long-term and non-linear, and anger, guilt, frustration and a sense of being trapped are common feelings (Remer and Elliott, 1988a).

While there is no clear end to the process, the secrecy that surrounds sexual abuse means there is no clear beginning either. In several cases, the women's relationships with their children had clearly been affected by the sexual abuse before they knew about it, although the exact date at which the abuse started was often still unknown. Both because pre-existing issues affected their response to the child's abuse and because the point at which the abuse started was often unclear, this section discusses the women's experience of mothering before, during and after the sexual abuse of their children.

The analysis presented here is informed by two central themes. First, in contrast to the view still prevalent in much psychological literature that mother–child bonding is natural and instinctive and provides automatic satisfaction in mothering, sociological research has indicated that the experience of mothering involves conflicts and contradictions that are rooted in the social conditions in which it is undertaken, and in which isolation, depression and frustration are common occupational hazards. The lack of other options for adult status and meaningful and rewarding work form the context in which mothering remains central to many women's identity over and above the actual relationship with children involved (Parton, C., 1990).

Second, while mothering can give a sense of meaning and purpose to women's lives, this is constructed by social interaction between the woman, her child and others and is consequently precarious. While the meaning accorded to mothering varies culturally and historically, one useful conceptualisation is offered by Boulton's (1983) study of women with pre-school children. Their sense of meaning and purpose related to three main factors: feelings of being needed and wanted, investment of hopes and dreams in children (including the desire to give their children better than the women had had themselves) and pride in the children (in which the judgements of others were important as well as their own) (Boulton, 1983). Although the present study involved children of varying ages, and the experience of mothering changes over the life course, Boulton's three factors were all recurring themes in the losses women described in relation to their children. The same study found women's experience of mothering was associated with the nature of their relationship with husbands, who were major sources of the women's view of themselves as mothers. Those without support from partners were more vulnerable to being overwhelmed by the everyday reality of unremitting child-care tasks and to losing all sense of meaning therein (Boulton, 1983), and have also been found to be more vulnerable to depression (Brown and Harris, 1978). Only two of the fifteen women in the present study could be said to have had a confiding relationship with their partners, and none of the women whose partners abused their children. However, the effects of this were mitigated for some by supportive relationships with family of origin and/or women friends.

While it was not possible clearly to separate pre-existing issues from effects of the abuse and accompanying disruption, there were two inter-related issues relevant to some (not all) of the women which were likely to have been continuous and which merit brief discussion: first, the over-investment of identity in mothering to the extent that in a minority of cases children were seen primarily as sources of nurturance for the mother rather than as individuals with separate needs, and, second (and more commonly), a sense of powerlessness and inability to influence events which resulted in overestimating children's capabilities.

A pattern of dependency on children to gratify the woman's own needs ('role reversal' as it is sometimes called) has been linked to women's experience of violence against themselves. Stark and Flitcraft (1988) suggest that where women are being assaulted themselves it represents their striving for selfhood and nurturance within the constraints of the mothering role. Where their options outside the home are severely restricted, children may be the only available source of nurturance. Over-investment of identity and dependency on children for the woman's own needs seemed to be an issue in five cases in this study (four involving abuse by partners and one sibling abuse), in three of which her partner was violent to the woman. In the two other cases, their husbands' absence due to work and drinking patterns, combined with relationships of conflict with families of origin, contributed to similar degrees of isolation from alternative sources of nurturance. In other cases too, and probably for all parents, there was some degree of expectation that children provide company and affection. However, supportive relationships with families of origin or adult women friends and meaningful work all lessened the likelihood of women over-investing their own needs in children.

Role reversal was in fact not an accurate representation of the way women saw their own relationships with children, except in one case in which the woman had always looked after her own mother and continued to do so, and expected her children to do the same for her. In seven of the eleven cases of father/father substitute abuse the women talked of their relationships with their children as involving mutually reciprocal expectations. The meaning of this clearly depends partly on the child's age – relating to an adolescent 'like sisters/friends' is different from doing so with a 6-year-old. However, there seemed to be two other sources of this in addition to the women's need for company and nurturance themselves. First, despite the objective power women had in relation to their children, which the majority expected to have and to entail responsibilities, many also expressed a subjective sense of powerlessness. This subjective sense of powerlessness to influence events in general, related to their own experiences of violence, isolation and consequent depression, meant they lacked confidence in their ability to exercise authority over their children and did not always recognise the latter's vulnerability in relation to adults. Second, a minority also expressed a reluctance to adopt an authoritative role, seeing this as inconsistent with their perspective on family life and/or child-rearing. To focus exclusively on powerlessness runs the risk of assuming a consensus on normal child-rearing practice which may obscure the different ideas of childhood and meanings involved in women's varying approaches to their roles as power-brokers between the wider society and their children.[1] One woman, for example, favoured a child-rearing style which minimised the guidance role of parents in the interests of children defining their own needs and desires.

These issues may be significant in increasing the child's vulnerability to abuse. However, they are also relevant background to the meaning of the abuse to the mother, since the losses involved are more devastating the more of her own identity is invested in the child, and the impact of the child's responses more threatening the less sense she has of her ability to influence them. A sense of powerlessness is also relevant to the difficulties some women had in defining behaviour as abuse (which rests above all on a recognition of the power relationship between adults and children).

It was difficult to identify clearly where problems caused by the abuse started since some women still did not know exactly when the abuse started and, where father/father substitute abuse was involved, the boundaries separating normal from abusive behaviour were often unclear. However, in seven cases, there seemed clear evidence that the abuse itself had contributed to problems with mothering before the women found out about it. In four cases, by the time they discovered the abuse, they had had periods of several years of unexplained difficulties with the child's behaviour, including severe sleeping problems, alternately hostile and demanding behaviour, lying and truanting. AN, for whom attendance at a child guidance clinic had made no difference, finally put the child's problems down to fate: 'I just thought she was an awkward customer.' PE, whose daughter had consistently complained of aches and pains, 'she had everything you didn't die of', for which no one could find any cause, attempted a number of strategies to improve the situation without success and concluded similarly: 'I thought she was taking the piss out of me.'

A history of unexplained difficulties prior to discovery undermined women's confidence in themselves as mothers, their pride in the child and their sense of being needed and wanted. This is not to suggest that, in the absence of abuse, family life is harmonious and conflict-free. Far from it – strong emotions and struggles for power are part of the everyday behaviour of children to their mothers (Walkerdine and Lucey, 1989). However, the survival skills children adopt to cope with sexual abuse add particular difficulties. These include 'hiding', 'acting out' and 'escaping' (running, fantasising or lying). Accounts of adult survivors suggest such responses are attempts to call attention to the fact that something is wrong, to escape their experience, or to mask it and their associated feelings of being different and bad from themselves and from others (Women's Research Centre, 1989). In addition, sexually abused children tend to behave with particular ambivalence towards their mothers, whether attempting to tell indirectly then retracting out of fear (Summit, 1983) or expressing anger and loss of trust at not being protected and/or guilt at their own involvement in keeping a secret (Scott and Flowers, 1988).

Where the abuser was their partner, the effects on their own relationship with the child were exacerbated by the interaction with him as well. In four cases, the abusive man had appeared to 'take over' the child, drawing her into the secrecy surrounding the abuse and excluding the mother. AN described this: 'They shut everybody out of everything.' PE, who felt her partner had set her daughter up as 'the woman of the house' in competition with her, described the effects of the secrecy on her own relationship with the child:

> Obviously me and K were growing further apart, he was putting her against me . . . it was getting to the point, if I told her off, they'd both sit there laughing at me, together. It was as if they'd sort of ganged up on me, sort of thing, and I couldn't say nothing to her any longer, without him intervening. He'd completely taken her over, he wouldn't even, if I bought her anything he used to get angry, and I just couldn't do nothing. (PE)

Children's descriptions of the victimisation process illustrate the way in which such 'special' relationships are constructed, with abusive men manipulating children's estrangement from potential sources of support (for example, threatening them with desertion by their mothers if they knew) as part of the process of 'grooming' the environment to ensure access (Berliner and Conte, 1990). Study of abusive men shows they are fully aware of this process and report targeting children for victimisation, systematically conditioning them to accept increasing sexual contact and exploiting the child's needs in order to maintain them as available victims (Conte *et al.*, 1989).

The sense of exclusion and rejection that the secrecy involves for mothers could comprise a loss in relation to one of the main sources of meaning and purpose in mothering where child care is seen as solely women's responsibility – that a child needs her mother more than anyone else (Boulton, 1983). While the older the child, the less she may be expected to have this exclusive primary relationship with her mother, the more she is expected to be responsible for her own behaviour so that actions which appear deliberately hostile and rejecting are more hurtful and undermining in the absence of understanding of their cause.

For three women, their response to their own exclusion involved conflict derived from a sense that mothering also entails fostering good father–child or stepfather–child relationships and the apparent closeness in the relationships was therefore partly a source of pride and pleasure to them (a further source of loss when its abusive nature was discovered). For one this undermined the legitimacy of her suspicions, which her partner dismissed as her jealousy. Another was particularly hurt in the aftermath by the twisting around in a custody battle of all her efforts to maintain the child's relationship with her father during the period of the abuse but before she knew about it.

The discovery of the sexual abuse entailed a sense of loss and regret that they had not known of it earlier for eleven of the fifteen women (despite in some cases their earlier ambivalence about finding out). Their sense of themselves as aware and protective mothers was threatened by the discovery and the inability of the child to tell them earlier implied the loss of her trust. For the two women who had been sexually abused by their own fathers as children and not been able to tell their mothers, and who had both had strong feelings about doing things differently for their own children, the child's inability to tell them, whether out of fear or desire to protect them, was particularly painful. The child's inability to tell (including denial when asked in several cases), entailed a hurtful loss of trust, to the extent of being experienced as deliberate deceit in one case. It also limited the mother's control and ability to find out what had happened and, where the child persisted in silence when questioned or only gradually 'admitted' further incidents, resulted in some anger and frustration for women. Those women who had most clearly come to terms with the child's loss of trust had understood it in terms both of the threats the abuser may have made to the child (including that her mother would kill her if she told in one case, that her mother would have her put in care in another) and also the difficulty of telling inherent in the experience of childhood sexual abuse. Two women felt their own experiences of sexual abuse as children (not by relatives), about which they had never told anyone, helped them to understand their children. As RD said, 'It's something you just don't talk about'. A third factor which was important in understanding their own previous lack of awareness was recognition of the abusive man's deliberate manipulation of the situation. For those women whom their children did tell, either spontaneously or on questioning, this provided an important vote of confidence in them, and for two retaining and rebuilding the child's trust was an important factor in sustaining their sense of meaning and purpose in the aftermath of discovery. As EJ put it:

> I sort of felt we were in this together . . . she totally relied on me to get it sorted out and somehow she knew that once I'd decided that I could do it, well I didn't, but she guided me you see. (EJ)

The threat to themselves as protectors of their children was more acute and induced more intense guilt for three women whose children had been abused or re-abused after they had known of other incidents by that man and therefore felt that they should have anticipated further incidents. None had done so at the time however, either because they had trusted the man's promises of reform or in one case because she had blocked out from conscious memory/'forgotten' the earlier incidents of abuse (her father's of her as a child).

For some the particular circumstances of the abuse added further losses. One woman felt worse because her child had been abused while she had been away training as a cub leader – hence she had been thinking of other children rather than her own. For three, guilt became attached to their being out at work when the abuse occurred and for two to their being asleep. For others, the fact that the child had been abused simply raised unspecific guilt about not being a good enough mother. One woman described her sense of guilt, 'I brought her into the world for this to happen' (AN). Another resisted the loss to her sense of self:

> I've not been a rotten mother, I can show you, I'll bring them to show you because I tell you what can't speak can't lie [showing photographs of children] . . . I mean look at the Christmases they've had, I've dressed up as Father Christmas and everything, there's been no reason. (LH)

Over-investment of identity in mothering was reflected in the intensity of these anxieties and the anticipation of blame from others. Particular ideas within this were important influences on response. One woman had clung to the idea that she would not allow her marriage to break up until all the children were eighteen. For another, treating all her children the same was central to her idea of herself as a mother and made the fact that she had had to accuse her son of abusing her daughter and then to choose between them devastating. While these ideas may have little relevance to the children's needs they are real sources of loss, threat and resistance to change for mothers.

In the aftermath several women expressed feelings of frustration, helplessness and inadequacy in relation to the effects on the child and their ability to help. Several made analogies with diseases or injuries where you knew more clearly what to do, such as the following example:

> Because I couldn't take, you know like if they're hurt you can get a plaster and something to wash the cut and put the plaster on it and after a while you watch that cut healing, now you've helped, you've actually done something. Or even if they've hurt their hand, I used to kiss it better, and they'd go away and they'd feel oh great, it might still be hurting them but mummy's kissed it better so because mummy's kissed it better everything's alright. So that, in that way I felt inadequate . . . as if I couldn't do anything to help her. (DK)

The difficulty of regaining the trust particularly of very young children exacerbated this sense of helplessness. In contrast one woman felt that once she knew what she had to do to help (leave her husband, which did in this case appear to resolve the child's problems), everything became easier: 'When you have to do something you just do it and hope that it'll work out all right don't you?' (EJ).

Four women found their children's anger and ambivalence towards them particularly distressing, although three of these felt that, given their knowledge of events at the time, they could not have done more than they had. KV commented, 'It's sad, frustrating, but I can't turn the clock back, I can't do anything about the past'. In another case the child's anger had been expressed in comparing her mother to the abusive stepfather, saying 'At least he loved me when he was doing that'. Her own anger at her ex-husband for his violence to her and to the child, as well as the ongoing threat to her mothering the child's anger posed, made this expression of the child's ambivalent feelings towards her stepfather too threatening for her to hear and she reacted angrily, 'He didn't love you, he hated you' (MG).

The sexually inappropriate behaviour of two young children (aged 6 and 7) caused acute embarrassment to their mothers in public, as well as heightening their anxiety about their risk of re-abuse. Children tend to be seen primarily as 'different from adults' (Backett, 1982) and protection from knowledge of sex is one of the ways this boundary is maintained (Ennew, 1986). Particularly with very young children, an obvious knowledge of sex (including the pregnancy of a 12-year-old girl) caused intense shame to their mothers, seeming to reflect on their ability to bring up children properly, as well as indicating losses for the children who were not ready for the 'knowledge' they had acquired. For some women their own lack of control about sex and the sense that 'natural' development had been disrupted seemed reflected in a sense of inevitability that the child was 'ruined for life' and might become promiscuous, withdraw from men, become a lesbian or otherwise be 'abnormal'. The long-term hopes invested in family often involve children, especially daughters, marrying and having children of their own (Backett, 1982; Boulton, 1983) and these possibilities represented real losses to the mother as well as, for some, fears that they would indicate harm to the child. These are well-documented long-term effects. However, they are by no means universal or inevitable, and both enabling children to tell sooner and improved support for them when they do may well reduce their incidence in the future. Moreover, Kelly's (1988a) reconceptualisation of such consequences as coping strategies which may have positive meaning is a useful corrective to the fears attached to them, as would be any lessening of the centrality of heterosexuality and marriage to women's identity.

For some children, the abuse had resulted in the adoption of an adult role, threatening the mothers' sense of being needed and wanted, and making them uncertain about their own role. In one case the child had clearly been set up in competition with her mother (PE) as the 'woman of the house' and the aftermath involved the mother reasserting herself as the adult and the child as the child, a change that was not achieved without conflict. As Roberts (1988) notes, girls given this position of 'power' are sometimes reluctant to give it up. In two other cases, much younger children (aged 6 and 7) had started to act, as one woman said, 'as an adult in a child's body' which both of their mothers found extremely difficult. Given that these women had little confidence in their ability to influence their children or events in general, the effects on the child, where they involved loss of trust in the mother, anger and adultified and sexually inappropriate behaviour, were ongoing sources of threat, and both women had developed some ways of coping by distancing these effects. One compared her daughter's behaviour to a horror film, the other described her child as 'weird . . . like an elderly person gone senile' (MG). To illustrate the difficulties that may be involved for mothers in the aftermath, it is worth quoting one account (AN's) at some length. The child concerned was sexually abused by her father from the age of 18 months to 5 years old without her mother's knowledge. Her behaviour had been difficult to cope with before her father left the home but afterwards, when AN had found out that sexual abuse had occurred, it became worse, partly it seemed because of the threats made to the child of what her mother would do to her if she told:

> She wasn't sleeping, she was awake all the time. I was passing out with anxiety. I was having actual blackouts, and she was standing over me. She looked worried when I came round, but as soon as she knew I was all right, she'd laugh. She would run from one room to the other at night time and I'd go to pick her up and cuddle her and she'd run away again to another corner. Then she'd run after me if I walked away from her, mummy mummy, and I'd go round to pick her up to comfort her and she'd run away in a corner again like an animal, eyes rolling in her head . . . .
>
> I can't take her to a swimming pool, because she's at level with a male's penis, in height. She can go with other people and she can just about bear it, but she won't go with me. Or if she goes with me, she's usually sick in the water, I have to take her out, she's screaming . . . she's very aware of men, she always looks at them, you know what she's thinking, she knows what's underneath their trousers and what happens with it . . . she shouldn't even be thinking like that at her age. (AN)

The child had gone into care with foster parents to give her mother a break but on her return eighteen months later, her behaviour was still difficult and involved constant reminders:

> She will not leave you alone until you answer every demand . . . She sends me I love you notes, tells everyone I'm her mummy . . . she goes on about when I was a baby, says 'I wish I was a baby and I could start all over again' . . . then she gets angry and says 'You had me, you've got to put up with me, do I look like him?' (AN)

Other people, including a police officer involved in the investigation of abuse, had expressed horror at the child's behaviour and AN was constantly aware that she stood out amongst other children.. In addition, her behaviour became worse when her mother had male company. In this context mothering brought little meaning and purpose, although her sense of guilt and duty meant she expressed resentment only reluctantly: 'The kid's trying hard, but what's there left for me?'

A further difficulty for this woman and two others was the sense that the child behaved very similarly to the abusive man. This perception is sometimes put down to transference but may well be an actual result of the process of 'taking over' the child involved in some abusive relationships. It was an added source of reminders and difficulties for women in the aftermath.

Older children were less likely to show the effects of their abuse in such overt fashion. It is possible that the older the child the more she may feel guilt at having kept the secret rather than anger at not being protected, and may be more inclined to withdraw rather than express her feelings. Given the sense that a child's well-being reflects on the mother (and the more so the younger the child), there is a strong incentive for women to believe their children are 'over it' if they are not showing overt signs. This is likely to be one reason why women are sometimes reluctant to involve their children in therapy or resistant to social work follow-up. It may also inhibit women from encouraging their children to talk about it (as well as dilemmas over the appropriate balance between 'bringing it out' and 'letting her forget' to resume normality). For those women whom the children continued to talk to about the abuse, it was an important indicator of their trust and therefore of restoring their sense of themselves as mothers, although it also meant ongoing reminders. Pride in their children was restored largely by the sense that they were more or less 'over it' and doing well. For one woman, the fact that the child was now happy as an adult and had an apparently good heterosexual relationship released her from guilt: 'It doesn't make me feel as though I must have done something dreadful for this to have happened to my daughter' (EJ). Two emphasised how dramatically their daughters had changed when the abusive men left the house, from being quiet, withdrawn and isolated to apparently confident and popular children. Three women with more sense of their ability to influence events than others had responded by working hard to rebuild their own relationships with the children in the aftermath. For these three women, the fact that the abuse had eventually resulted in closer relationships between them and their daughters than they had had previously gave it some positive meaning. As one said, 'Assume you can change everything' (EJ).

This section has outlined the women's experience of secondary victimisation, that is, the way in which the sexual abuse of their children affected their relationships with them, and detailed some of the sources of variation within this. All the women described some losses in this context, whatever the relationship of the perpetrator of abuse to them. For those whose relationship to the perpetrator had been a close one – as partner, father or son – there were further losses, equally long term, in that context. The next section focuses on only one of the ways in which their relationship with the abusive man affected their experience at the time of the child's abuse, as a source of their own primary victimisation.

PRIMARY VICTIMISATION

For women whose children were sexually abused by their partners, it was important to understand the meaning of the child's abuse to them within the overall pattern of marital violence, conflict and control within which it occurred. Discussion of the violence of incest perpetrators towards their wives has tended to focus on the high incidence of domestic violence in the marital relationship (Dietz and Craft, 1980; Truesdell *et al.*, 1986; Gordon, 1989). However there is a far wider range of forms of control which operate, including psychological and sexual violence, and a number of sites of conflict including money, sexuality, reproduction and child-rearing. This section will focus primarily on sexual violence, adopting Kelly's definition which includes:

> any physical, visual, verbal or sexual act that is experienced by the woman or girl, at the time or later, as a threat, invasion or assault, that has the effect of hurting her or degrading her and/or takes away her ability to control intimate contact.

> (Kelly, 1988a, p. 41)

Within this definition, the sexual abuse of a child by the mother's partner may be conceptualised as itself a form of sexual violence against the mother, as well as being commonly accompanied by other forms of control.

In nine of the eleven cases of father/father substitute abuse, the mother had been victimised physically, verbally and/or sexually herself. Although of these the two women still living with abusive partners minimised the problems, in all these relationships the men had dominated, although with varying patterns of control and varying forms of resistance from the women. In the two remaining cases the women regarded themselves as the dominant partners and reported no incidents of direct violence against themselves. However, although the latter two women, unlike most of the others, had not been physically in fear of their partners, for both the sexual abuse of their daughters had a coercive and humiliating meaning for them in the context of marital relationships in which they had little sense of their own right to control sexual contact.

All eleven women were aware that men's right of sexual access was part of the traditional marital bargain, and had been subjected to some form of sexual pressure. This ranged from rape, attempted rape and various forms of coercion to the feeling that sex was primarily a duty rather than a matter of choice, lack of knowledge about sexuality as well as ideas about marriage contributing to their lack of control more than specific use of force. Of the two cases in which the women regarded themselves as the dominant partner, one had not known how she became pregnant the first time and the other felt that sex was not particularly important to her but felt 'abnormal' because of its idealised cultural significance and threatened by her husband's expressions of sexual interest in women he saw on television, for instance.

Kelly (1988a) found that women wanting non-coercive heterosexual relationships defined these as involving the ability to say no to sex without negative consequences. This involves challenging dominant definitions of marriage which still accord men rights of sexual access (Pateman, 1988)[2] and none of these women could be said to have had such non-coercive relationships. Two women had submitted to incessant sexual demands from their husbands for the sake of peace. Others who had resisted expressed guilt at 'not giving him enough', if they had not wanted sex as often as their partners did, although in three cases it was their partners who had apparently lost interest in sex with them. Only one woman expressed a clear sense of having a right to control her own sexual contact and no guilt or ambivalence about resisting her husband's pressure. In the absence of this sense of sexual autonomy and in the context of various forms of pressure in their own sexual relationships, their partner's sexual abuse of a child, especially a teenage daughter, contributed to pressure on them, either directly or indirectly, and hence was experienced as a form of violence against themselves.

Directly, in four cases, the behaviour women witnessed during periods of suspicion appeared to involve using the child partly for a visual assault/ threat against them. KV, for example, observed her husband's suggestive remarks to her daughter, made in front of her, within the context of a pattern of sexual violence against herself which involved forcing certain practices on her which she did not like, nagging her while she sat up all night in resistance if she did not want sex, undermining her confidence with accusations regarding her sexual hang-ups and talking to friends about their sex life in front of her. Her hurt and fear at this behaviour led to her withdrawing further from sexual contact with her husband and consequently increased nagging from him. His behaviour to the child, which included telling the child (in KV's absence) that her mother would not let him have sex with her, and (in her presence) wanting to buy the child nice underwear when they went shopping or making suggestive remarks to the child when he saw a woman he fancied on television were further incidents in this pattern. She described this as 'he treated her like he should have treated me, that's what made me feel uncomfortable'. This induced not jealousy, but feelings of loss of control and humiliation.

As well as the apparently deliberate use of the child by the abuser to humiliate the mother by setting her up in sexual competition, less direct pressure was experienced by women who had not witnessed suspicious behaviour but who on discovering the abuse adopted the common-sense (and false) 'he can't have been getting enough elsewhere' explanation and consequently suffered guilt about their own sexual relationships if there had been any pre-existing problems. Many sexually abusive men engage in sexual activity obsessively, with their wives and children (and often others outside the family) concurrently (Herman and Hirschman, 1981b; Faller, 1988b). In addition, where sexual frustration is an issue, there are always other options for resolving it, such as masturbation.

A related issue in the patterns of control and resistance was control over fertility and reproduction. Kelly (1988a) has noted that domestic violence may involve both forced pregnancy and attempts to terminate pregnancy (by battering directed at the womb area for instance). Two cases in the present study suggested the relevance of this to the sexual abuse of the child. In both, the mother's decision not to have another child was followed by the sexual abuse of a daughter resulting in pregnancy and childbirth. In one of these cases the woman's husband had threatened her in previous fights over whether to have another child that he would go out and get one and she would have to look after it. She scoffed at this threat at the time but this had in fact been the result of the abuse of the child.

In all the cases of abuse by partners, the abuse of the child had implications for women's own sense of control. In the nine cases in which their husbands dominated the women directly as well as via their child's abuse, violence to the mother preceded the abuse of the child. This did not mean that the women passively submitted to the child's abuse to relieve themselves as has sometimes been argued. Violence to themselves usually continued alongside the abuse of the child, which represented an extension of control rather than a transfer. Abuse of the child did seem in some cases to be a response to the man's control over the woman slipping as her strength or resistance increased. In one case the sexual abuse of the child started shortly after the woman had gone back to full-time work, to which her partner had agreed for financial reasons but which threatened his control, although he continued to reassert it over her every evening. In another, the woman expressed relief when her partner decided to leave, some time after the discovery of his sexual abuse, to which his response was to throw the child across the room.

Children were used by violent men both to extend means of control over their mothers (for example by battering or verbally undermining women in the presence of children as well as by sexually abusive behaviour) and to extend their domain of control to someone with less power to resist. This pattern has also been found to be common in relation to physical abuse of children (Stark and Flitcraft, 1988; Bowker *et al.*, 1988). It indicates the need to understand women's responses to their children's victimisation in the context of their own experiences of primary victimisation as well as in relation to secondary victimisation.

Eight of the fifteen women in this study also reported incidents of sexual abuse from their own childhoods (under the age of 16), two by their fathers and the others by non-members of the household, memories of which had been triggered by their child's abuse. While mothers' own experience of sexual abuse in childhood is often used to support 'cycle of abuse' theories (see Goodwin *et al.*, 1981; Vizard and Tranter, 1988), this study found that the relevance of childhood to the meaning of their experience was broader, more complex and much less determined than cycle of abuse arguments suggest. The next section describes the significance of childhood in their ability to come to terms with the losses their child's abuse entailed. Here it is relevant to note that the women's own experience of childhood sexual abuse could be a resource on which they drew to understand their children's experience, but could also be an extra source of guilt. Despite their lack of objective validity, cycles have a subjective appeal in the 'why me? why her?' stage (Janoff-Bulman and Frieze, 1983) of coming to terms with loss. This appeal carries strong risks, particularly where the guilt often felt by women who have been sexually abused as children is still unresolved. DK who had been abused by her own father as a child and whose daughter was abused by a cousin when baby-sitting, described this:

I thought to myself why the hell did I have my children, why did god let this happen to them, you know, why should my children be abused, why should somebody try to hurt her when she'd never tried to hurt anybody. I also thought to myself well maybe it was something that I did in my life, something bad, you know really bad that I'd done and she was being punished for it . . . all sorts of things went through my mind, I thought perhaps that it was because of when my father was abusing me, there were times when I actually enjoyed it . . . all these things went through my mind. (DK)

THE LOSS MODEL

Both secondary victimisation and primary victimisation involve loss and a grieving process was a central theme in the women's accounts. This section discusses factors which may influence women's ability to come to terms with the losses, and offers an alternative way of understanding responses which have often been labelled collusion. The grieving that loss induces is a process which has to be worked out – from shock through acute distress to reintegration (Marris, 1986). Doing so involves reconciling the conflicting impulses (to return to the time before the loss occurred and to reach forward to a state of mind where the loss is forgotten) by extracting from the past its meaning for the present. Marris suggests four kinds of conditions which may affect the ability to reconstitute meaning, which were relevant to this study.

First, the person's own experience of attachment in childhood may influence their general sense of security and resilience in the face of loss. Studies of mothers' responses, influenced by the appealing symmetry of cycle of abuse theories, tend to focus on whether the mother was sexually abused herself as a child, and have found no significance in relation to different responses (Myer, 1984; de Jong, 1988; Gomes-Schwartz *et al.*, 1990), although there is some evidence that mothers who were sexually abused themselves suffer increased stress (Kelley, 1990). The present study suggests that childhood experience may have a broader relevance, affected by the stage the mother has reached in resolving it. Those women who had most difficulty in resolving their loss were not those who reported being sexually abused themselves, but those who retained idealised images of their childhoods despite accounts which indicated considerable conflict. This analysis is consistent with Egeland *et al.* (1988) who found that women who were aware of their own past history of abuse and how it had affected them were less likely to have child care problems later than those who were not.

The centrality of loss to the experience of mothers of sexually abused children suggests that if a cycle exists it may be of quite a different order to that thought to operate for other forms of abuse. The evidence to support all cycle of abuse theories is considerably less convincing than often suggested (Burgess and Youngblade, 1988; Widom, 1989). The impact of childhood abuse on later life is mediated by many factors. However, if explanations for 'intergenerational transmission' are offered in terms of learning that violence is appropriate or acceptable in families (Shields and Hanneke, 1988), this is clearly inappropriate to women whose children are sexually abused in their absence and who are unable to accept that this has happened.

Second, the more conflicted, doubtful or unresolved the meaning of what has been lost, the harder it is likely to be to reconstitute meaning in a way which successfully disengages emotion and purpose from irretrievable circumstances. The uncertainty surrounding definition, explanation and long-term implications expressed by several women, and the common uncertainty of circumstances in which the abuse took place and at some stages the identity of the abuser must all inhibit mothers from resolving their own sense of loss and discontinuity. Two women described their feelings when suspicion shifted from one member of the family to another in fairly similar terms, as 'like we're falling apart here, everything was being destroyed'.

Third, the less opportunity people have to prepare for a loss, and the less predictable and meaningful the event itself, the more traumatically the whole structure of meaning will be disrupted and the more insecure all attachment thereafter will seem. For only one woman in this study was her husband's abuse of her child at all predictable. Although a cumulative process of discovery provided some staggering of disruption, those who discovered abuse in the family suddenly could be faced with the disruption of all closest attachments at once, by an event for which all the cultural images of marriage and family give no preparation. Those women who knew their partners were violent in other ways, however, seemed to find it easier to come to terms with the abuse than those who had previously thought their marriages happy.

Fourth, events after the loss may either support the process of recovery, encouraging the ambivalent impulses loss induces to work themselves out, or frustrate it. Women in this study were rarely given the opportunity to work through their own ambivalence in either informal or formal contacts, but were usually faced immediately with instructions, expectations set by others and often disbelief or blame (see Chapters 6 and 7). Those who had become stuck in unresolved grief bore particularly vivid memories of the negative responses of others, and tended to have felt totally isolated, faced with conflict and secrecy within the family and blame and instructions from outside.

As noted above, grieving is a process, and the sources of loss multiple and ongoing. Hence it is not easy to draw a clear boundary around the resolving of all loss, and some aspects remained unresolved for most women. In particular, the sense of betrayal by abusive men was a source of ongoing anger and bitterness which several felt was the most difficult and unrecognised aspect of their experience. For two, their own experiences of violence from the child's abuser remained unresolved, aspects of them still being unspeakable, after they had to some extent come to terms with the child's abuse.

The centrality of loss suggests an alternative way of understanding responses that have often been labelled collusive, that is, failing to prevent further abuse once suspicions have arisen. These were in some cases better represented as a mixture of resistance and accommodation to the particular threats or losses involved, to the women's sense of femininity, identity as mothers and so on. Breakwell (1986) notes that, when identity is threatened, coping strategies are adopted which either deflect or accept the threat. Acceptance is rarely wholesale capitulation however, rather reflecting a compromise negotiated between the threat and the needs of identity for continuity, distinctiveness and self-esteem.

One woman's response illustrates this process, involving a struggle to preserve what was important to her and, at the same time, to deflect the threat the abuse represented via coping strategies such as denial, repression and minimisation. LH, whose husband abused her teenage daughter in the context of a relationship which she defined as a love affair between them, alternately pushed her suspicions to the back of her mind and confronted them both, in the hope of obtaining proof with which she could stop it. She also alternated between ensuring her husband had clean clothes and cigarettes when she was in and going out with other men in an attempt to restore her self-esteem. When her daughter became pregnant and had a child – and both husband and daughter continued to deny her accusations that he was the father – she redefined herself as the baby's mother. This went on for several years before she left, and she was aware that others would think she had condoned the abuse and adamant that she had not. A sense of powerlessness is an important influence on such responses but does not necessarily result in passive submission. Rather, where all available options seem likely to result in further negative consequences, minimising the effects on the child or blaming her ('she liked it/she was the seducer') redefines the situation as one not requiring protective action.

SUMMARY AND CONCLUSIONS

The sources of loss women face when a child is sexually abused are many, various and ongoing. Some of these derive from the woman's relationship with her child and comprise a form of secondary victimisation. Some of them derive from her relationship with the perpetrator, especially but not only if he is her partner. Others derive from the broader context of relationships within which the abuse occurs and of her own life. There is a sense in which child sexual abuse faces everyone who comes into contact with it with loss. Social workers also often cope with the emotional impact of child sexual abuse by blocking out some or all of its aspects. This occurs even in training sessions, where no direct relationship with a child who has been sexually abused or a perpetrator of abuse is involved.[3] The personal stress engendered by direct work has been described as 'impossible to over-estimate' (Pringle, 1990, p. 23).

Two cautionary notes regarding the use of the loss model with women whose children are sexually abused are in order. It is not intended to imply either that all mothers' reactions to child sexual abuse are loss related or that all their losses are child sexual abuse related. The danger of making the first assumption is indicated by the observation of disabled people that an understanding of responses to disability as loss-related is sometimes used by others to deny the legitimacy of their anger at oppressive social conditions (Oliver, 1983). There is a similar danger that women's anger at sexual violence, at the difficulties mothers face in protecting their children, and at the responses of public agencies, may be interpreted as grief to be worked through personally, rather than a response to conditions requiring social change. The second point is that, while the discovery of child sexual abuse involves a specific and new threat, mothering can be seen as a 'state of perpetual coping', characterised by constant demands and disruptions, at least in its early stages (Graham, 1982). Indeed, there is evidence that coping strategies such as denial are not uncommon even before mothering begins, in young women's responses to pregnancy (Wilczynski, 1991). The danger here is that other important aspects of women's experience may be overlooked if child sexual abuse is assumed to be the trigger to all loss. One study found no significant difference in levels of depression between mothers of sexually abused children and mothers of non-abused children attending an out-patient clinic for psychological evaluation (Wagner, 1991). This is likely to be due to both the high levels of depression common in women with young children (Brown and Harris, 1978) and the variability of experience within both groups.

Nevertheless, the significance of loss in women's responses to child sexual abuse suggests a number of factors which may influence them.

Women are likely to resolve the grieving process more easily if they have had secure experiences of attachment as a child themselves and/or opportunities to compensate for deficits via non-abusive relationships later,[4] if they have an understanding of sexual abuse, its roots and implications generally, if the circumstances and nature of the child's abuse are known and if they are prepared in some way for it by their knowledge of the perpetrator. They are also likely to resolve the losses more easily if their own experiences of and responses to loss are validated by others in the aftermath, and time is allowed for them to work through the conflicting impulses of resistance and adaptation that grief involves. As Remer and Elliott put it, 'the secondary victim *must* feel supported and understood to be able to comprehend and let in the experience of the primary victim; a difficult, frustrating and sometimes threatening task' (1988b, p. 393). Care needs to be taken not to exacerbate the losses women already face. Attributing abuse by a partner to marital sexual problems, for example, reinforces the lack of control over their own sexuality which women commonly feel already. Attributing it to their partner's search for eternal youth (a popular form of psychoanalytic explanation) may further threaten their sense of femininity. Implicating women by their absence when the abuse occurred increases their feelings of guilt and may result in giving up paid work or friendships to stay home and thereby depleting their resources further. Emphasising the damage to the child and long-term effects in an attempt to impress the seriousness of it on mothers is likely to exacerbate their existing fears.

Rather, maintaining and increasing women's psychological, social and economic resources is vital. Continuity in areas of life not directly affected is an important factor in coming to terms with loss. Women develop more positive ways of coping as their sense of their ability to influence events increases, and hence the need to forget or redefine events is reduced. Their own experiences of victimisation need to be recognised and their own right to sexual autonomy and physical safety emphasised as well as the child's. A clear statement of the abuser's sole accountability for the sexual abuse needs to be made. Perhaps most important is to identify what women can do to reduce the impact of abuse on the child, by informing them of the importance of their support to children's recovery and of the support to be made available to them.

4 Finding out

The discovery process

Whether women know or not that their child is being sexually abused has been a key point of conflict in debates over the mother's role. Kempe and Kempe (1978), for example, argued in the past that mothers always knew about abuse in the family at some level. It is now recognised that they often do not, since the abuse usually occurs in their absence and children are commonly sworn to secrecy, threatened with harm to themselves and/or their mother if they tell. Children often make great efforts not to let their mothers know, and have complex and ambivalent feelings about others knowing, as well as wanting the abuse itself to stop. Children's resistance to telling derives mainly from fear of losing the affection or goodwill of the abuser and fear that they will be disbelieved, blamed or harmed. The less loyalty they feel to the offender, the more likely they are to tell, and they are least likely to tell when the abuser is a natural parent (Gomes-Schwartz *et al.*, 1990). Children often also believe their mothers know when they in fact do not.

The debate over women knowing or not about their children's abuse continues, however. Feminists have recently been criticised for implying that mothers never know (La Fontaine, 1990), and the question of knowledge is important in practice for two reasons. Social work assessment commonly involves establishing whether the mother knew or not, to determine whether she participated in or was unable to protect the child from abuse, and a central objective of social work intervention in the aftermath is ensuring that women do know and believe in order to protect their children from further abuse. This study started from the premise that, if women were not present at the time of the abuse, they must in some way find out about it, and sought to explore the process of discovery, to illuminate both the interactions within the family and the ways in which mothers may be helped to believe that abuse has taken place.

The term commonly used to describe the breaking of secrecy is 'disclosure' – a term which suggests a single point in time when all is revealed.

Women themselves talked of 'finding out', and described this in enormous detail, often with dates and times of day to locate particular incidents over a period of time, and reported confrontations and conversations with other people, within and outside the family. For some women there was a clearly identifiable point at which they found out about the abuse, but for others discovery was a cumulative process. Within this process they talked of not knowing, and why they felt they had not, of noticing that 'something was wrong' and of suspecting abuse but needing their suspicions confirmed. While the losses involved in the sexual abuse of a child meant that their motivation to find out fluctuated, even when attempting to confirm suspicions they were not always able to do so. Discovery is an active and interactive process which develops over time and has no clear beginning or end. Mothers are often presented only as disbelieving or as 'tuning out' signals, but some of the women interviewed had become preoccupied with attempts to discover what was happening, despite many obstacles to doing so, and to the exclusion of developing effective ways of protecting their children.

There are similarities with the handling and disclosure of other secrets, and Glaser and Straus's (1964) analysis, developed in relation to awareness of dying, spies, the gay community, the handling of stigmatised diseases and so on, is relevant here. Glaser and Straus adopt the concept of awareness contexts to summarise the total combination of what each interactant in a situation knows about the identity of the other and their own identity in the eyes of the other. At its simplest level, the identity of one person alone is at stake (e.g. a dying patient), but where two identities are involved (e.g. spy and counter-spy) it becomes more complex, and correspondingly more so the more actors are involved. Where two actors are involved, they suggest four types of awareness context, open (in which each is aware of the other's true identity), closed (in which one does not know the other's identity), suspicion (a modification of closed, in which one suspects the true identity of the other) and pretence (a modification of open in which both are fully aware but pretend not to be). The analysis focuses on the interactive process by which awareness contexts are maintained or transformed, according to the gains and losses to each actor.

It is useful to consider this model in relation to an example other than child sexual abuse to illustrate the way in which the combination of sex, stigma and fear can lead to distorted patterns of communication (rather than, as is often argued, communication difficulties resulting in sexual abuse). There are similarities, for instance, with the process involved in adult children coming out (or not) as gay or lesbian to their parents. This often involves testing tactics on both sides (dropping hints, leaving books around and so on to test the waters), complex combinations of who knows what and who believes who else does and does not know (which may be correct or not) and pressure from heterosexual siblings to protect parents from the information. This sort of pattern can go on for years without open communication between all members ever being established, although movement towards it may occur if testing tactics get a favourable response or motivation is increased by, for example, the access of a lover during illness being at issue. Alternatively, it can become more difficult to reveal the secret, as the longer things have been left unsaid the more there is to reveal and the guilt for the 'child' at having kept the secret is added to the other problems (Baetz, 1984; Muller, 1987; Markowe, 1990). In many ways this should be an easier secret to reveal than a child's of sexual abuse. Adults are no longer dependent on their parents for survival, and the information is considerably less likely to break up the parents' marriage. Nevertheless, parents commonly suffer a bereavement-like response to children coming out (Muller, 1987) and in both cases there is a sense that there is little to be gained by the parents in acquiring this information. The social rewards of both positions are limited.

The interaction surrounding sexual abuse by a family member is equally if not more complicated. In the present study, children had both thought their mothers knew when they did not and thought they did not know when they did. Siblings had sometimes been told first and contributed to silencing the child, in one case getting the abused child's pocket money off her in exchange for keeping the secret. Children attempted to tell in highly indirect ways and sometimes lashed out angrily at their mothers when questioned. Women who became suspicious also often questioned children indirectly – feeling awkward about asking a direct question. Women often missed the hints that their children dropped, which were open to a wide variety of interpretations and only became defined as hints in retrospect. Even such an apparently obvious one as 'Why don't you divorce daddy?' (and most were less direct, more along the lines of 'Can I come to the launderette with you?') is not necessarily indicative of the child being abused where the mother is also being subjected to violence. Women who suspected the child was being abused then had to assess who was the likely abuser, and in several cases more than one possible abuser was involved in the process. Women both pretended not to know once they did in order to avoid violent repercussions while working out a response and pretended to know more than they did in order to confirm suspicions. Men questioned about abuse sometimes denied consistently and at other times confessed, pleading remorse and promising reform to prevent the information going further.

This chapter, after an initial section on the timing and pattern of the mothers' discovery processes, is structured around the awareness contexts most common in the women's accounts – closed, suspicion and open, as these relate to their knowledge of the child's experience of abuse. They are referred to however in the terms women themselves used – not knowing, suspecting and knowing, which emphasise the dynamic interactions and negotiations that occur within each level of awareness and the process of change. Because of the number of individuals involved, and the other issues to be known (the mother's awareness of who is the abuser, the abuser's and the child's awareness of what the mother's awareness is and so on), there are a number of different combinations of awareness covered within each section. However, they are grouped like this for simplicity and to represent the sense of a process of discovery which mothers described. Within each, there are issues concerning what kind of information is involved, the visibility, accessibility and interpretation of information, the evaluation of it, and convincing relevant others about the interpretation of information, which are common to all awareness phenomena (Straus, 1987).

Within this analysis there are three ways in which the interaction surrounding child sexual abuse is different from that surrounding many secrets. First, the key actors are all interacting within one of the primary arenas in which an individual's reality is constructed, the family. Hence, there is considerable potential for confusion and for the manipulation of reality by abusers through control of information as well as of other resources. Even without the secrecy surrounding child sexual abuse, women abused themselves by partners are not always aware of it at the time, since the emotional abuse underlying all forms of violence involves a distortion of subjective reality which undermines their faith in their own perceptions (Kirkwood, 1991). A common defence mechanism is also to identify (at least to some extent) with the abuser's world view in order to ensure survival (Graham *et al.*, 1988). As Berger and Luckman put it, 'he who has the bigger stick has the better chance of imposing his definitions of reality' (1967, p. 127). The losses involved for women in the discovery of a child's sexual abuse, combined with the dominance and violence of the majority of the abusers, made the sustaining of an independent reality difficult. On top of this, there is a moral significance attached to families being 'worlds of their own' and parents being a 'united front' (Ribbens, 1990). Women are expected and commonly expect themselves to play a particular role in sustaining these shared realities. Women faced with conflicting versions of events and their meaning therefore attempted, to varying degrees, to mediate – to reconcile the conflicts between the accounts of others, and between these and their own perceptions.

Second, some specific problems of communication arise in the discovery of child sexual abuse. Children may not be capable of communicating about the abuse, because of their age and/or their attempts to mask the reality from themselves as well as others. As Summit (1988) has argued, and many workers have found, even if children are listened to carefully, much of their reality may be missed. Depression in both mother and child may also lead to low levels of communication about anything (Levang, 1988), and the denial and devaluation of female experience, both generally and within families, may inhibit mothers from hearing and validating their daughters' realities in particular (Miller, 1990).

Third, while the definition of some forms of secret behaviour may be self-evident, the definition of sexual abuse is not. 'Abuse' is by definition wrong but for the most part women are observing behaviour and relationships which form a continuum, and which do not come clearly labelled as 'normal' or 'abusive'. Victimised children too have described the process of sexualisation as a gradual one with no clearly identifiable point at which the relationship changed from normal to sexual (Berliner and Conte, 1990; Gomes-Schwartz *et al.*, 1990). The problem of definition is not exclusive to sexual abuse. Definitions of physical abuse of children are not self-evident and vary considerably between professionals. Women's definitions of their own experience of violence are similarly complex. In both circumstances, physical injury and perceptions of the abuser's intention are key criteria (Herzberger and Tennen, 1988; Sedlak, 1988). The problem of definition in relation to child sexual abuse is compounded however both by the inaccessibility of information about events conducted in secrecy and the common invisibility of harm. As well as their resistance to telling, sexually abused children do not always show behavioural signs that indicate the need for some intervention (Gomes-Schwartz *et al.*, 1990), let alone that give clear indication of sexual abuse. Sources of confusion over the evaluation of events once they are known are discussed in the last section of the chapter, 'Knowing'. However, the confusion expressed over what exactly constitutes sexual abuse is clearly a factor affecting all stages of the discovery process.

TIMING AND PATTERN

The process of discovery is difficult to chart accurately in retrospect for two reasons. First, the mother's awareness and understanding have usually been changed through and by the process. Once women know, the fact that they have not known before becomes problematic, and is often a source of guilt, hindering clarity of memory. There is no way of clearly defining a correct or appropriate level of awareness. Although a high level of awareness or suspicion depends partly on political consciousness (Campbell, 1988), it also involves a loss of trust and it is likely that most women would be reluctant to suspect and monitor those close to them beyond a certain extent. Where that line is drawn varies and discussing why it appears that some women did not know for perhaps longer than would be expected therefore involves making somewhat arbitrary and subjective distinctions.

Second, and related to this, it is not always clear in retrospect which observations seemed evidence of abuse or 'something wrong' at the time, and which have new meaning as such in the light of current knowledge. As Campbell wrote of the police response to evidence of sexual abuse, 'evidence is not neutral, nor does it fall from the sky: it has to be discovered. Detection is an ideological endeavour to make sense of a mystery' (1988, p. 78). The loss and confusion accompanying women's discovery of a child's sexual abuse means that the attempt to make sense often takes years, and past evidence is repeatedly reinterpreted through current consciousness. Reported actions taken, such as confrontations and strategies for obtaining proof, can be taken as clear indicators of suspicion at the time, however.

Discovery can take several years (a cumulative discovery) or it can be collapsed into minutes (a sudden discovery). It may involve the mother and child only or more commonly a range of others, both within and outside the family, whose involvement may act as validation or as further obstacles to overcome. It may involve a period of not knowing about the abuse, followed by a period of suspecting followed by a period of knowing or one or both of the first two stages may be omitted if the mother finds out fairly quickly after the abuse starts. The process is interwoven both with the woman's own response to loss and with decisions taken about family relationships and is therefore not a straightforward linear one. Although there are distinctions between not knowing, suspecting and knowing, which are not adequately addressed by the concept of denial, the boundaries between these phases are often blurred. In particular, the transition between not knowing and suspecting (feeling that 'something was wrong') seemed to belong sometimes in 'not knowing' and sometimes in suspecting, depending on whether and how consistently abuse was considered as a possible explanation for the available evidence.

For twelve of the fifteen women in this study, the abuser was living in the household with the child at the time of the abuse. Of these twelve, eight women did not know about the abuse for a substantial period of time, ranging from less than a year to over five years. Of these eight, three then became suspicious, one taking a year, another two years before their suspicions were confirmed and the third never quite confirming her suspicions about an ongoing relationship between father and daughter (the latter now in her 20s) which both denied to her yet persisted in while she eventually moved out of the house. The other five found out in a sudden clearly identifiable incident, although that was often followed by a period of reassessment and confirmation and for one, recurring confusion and ambivalence which remained unresolved three years later. One of these five described a feeling of something wrong before finding out, and two others described previous problems in the family but for which they had had other interpretations. Two of the women who found out in a sudden incident were those who decided to stay or reunite with their partners later. For one, when the abuse recurred (within a year), she knew; for the other, when it started again (three years after the first discovery), she did not know, and only after three more years felt that something was wrong and after a further year found out.

Three women became suspicious shortly after the abuse started, one taking over a year and another four years before those suspicions were confirmed. The third appeared to have waited for proof without actively pursuing it, and for her the boundary between suspecting and knowing was less clear. One woman knew of her husband's behaviour (touching his children's genitals) as it occurred, although she was not present at the particular incident which triggered her definition of it as abuse. Even for her however, there was a form of discovery process, involving a re-evaluation of the information she had in order to define it as abuse, a process which was still continuing at the time of the interview.

There were also three cases in this study where the abuser was a relative but not within the household. Two of the mothers found out when the child said something which indicated abuse to them, one to a sibling (three years after the first incident of abuse, but shortly after the second separate incident), the other to her mother's cohabitee (a week after the first incident of abuse). The third did not know that her child was being abused on visits to his grandfather over a period of four years, although she put a stop to the visits as soon as the child said he no longer wanted to go there. She found out only two years after the visits were stopped.

NOT KNOWING

How is it possible for a child to be sexually abused by a member of the household or close relative without the mother knowing or suspecting? This section discusses the accounts of women whose partners abused their children while living with them and one whose father (the child's grandfather) abused her son over four years on visits to his house. Although the selection of cases where the mother had not known for longer than might be expected is somewhat arbitrary, they themselves all saw their not knowing as problematic, as a source of guilt (to varying degrees) and something that they needed to understand and explain. In fact, at the time of the interviews, the majority of the women still did not know the full details of what had happened.

The degree of awareness the women had had that 'something was wrong' for their children varied, both between women and over time. In addition, the information available from both the children and the partners/father was limited and open to a variety of interpretations. None of the children had told directly during this time, and some had denied anything was wrong when asked. This is a common pattern. Summit (1983) has developed a five-stage model of children's response to sexual abuse (the child sexual abuse accommodation syndrome) which involves i) secrecy, ii) helplessness, iii) entrapment and accommodation, iv) delayed, conflicted and unconvincing disclosure and v) retraction. As he points out, the patterns of behaviour commonly involved in children's attempts to cope with and maintain the secrecy imposed on them commonly lead to them being discredited as 'impossible' before they even attempt to tell.

In most cases, the women had been aware of some problems for their children but had not considered sexual abuse as a possible explanation. One had put her child's 'precociousness' at school and insomnia down to pre-existing health problems since the child had always been very small and was bullied by children at school because of this. Another attributed her daughter's nervous and withdrawn behaviour variously to unhappiness at school, the effects of poor housing and to herself being out at work. Two women attributed vaginal soreness in their children to urinary problems or not wiping themselves properly, and one attributed her child's distress on being left at nursery, and quiet, withdrawn behaviour there, as due to her wearing glasses. Two attributed their daughters' fear of their husbands to having witnessed violence against themselves and to the normality of fear of him in the household. Three however perceived their daughters' relationships with their husbands as unusually close, and either felt pleased at this or that they should be. The suspicion of sexual abuse does not come quickly. To some extent, these interpretations indicate the unthinkableness of incestuous abuse, particularly at a time when there was no public recognition of its existence though it is still a factor in relation to people's own families now. The belief in personal invulnerability is one of the basic assumptions that victimisation shatters (Janoff-Bulman and Frieze, 1983). These interpretations also however represent plausible (and possibly more likely) explanations for what the mother has observed.

The behaviour of the abusive men was also confusing and, while in retrospect seemed to indicate sexual abuse, was subject to a variety of other interpretations at the time. PE attributed her partner's unpredictable behaviour to her daughter (sometimes 'the perfect father', sometimes seeming not to like her) to his personality since he behaved similarly to her. When he encouraged her to go out, offering to look after the child in her absence, she felt lucky and was reinforced by friends in doing so. When he lost interest in their sexual relationship, telling her he no longer loved her, she assumed there was 'another woman'. And when he told her that if it was not for her daughter he would leave, 'I used to interpret that as like a father with his children, it's only for the children keeping us together type of thing'.

While the tactics abusers employed to maintain secrecy and the ambivalence of the children about others knowing meant that evidence was not easily accessible and what there was was open to various interpretations, the mothers' accounts also suggested the need to understand their own levels of awareness. The most common factor which seemed significant in reduced awareness was their own experience of violence, either current or past, but lack of confidence in their own parenting and low expectations of family life also contributed.

For five women, fear of their partners was a part of daily life and the costs of confrontation included violence to the extent of hospitalisation and threats of murder. Hence they were preoccupied with ways of coping, resisting and surviving themselves (Kelly, 1988a) which reduced their awareness of and availability to their children. MG talked of the way she 'switch[ed] everything off, just switch my mind off' to cope both with her husband raping her repeatedly and with the incessant demands of three children under five. RD watched out for signs of her husband's violence and attempted to hurt him (verbally) first or walked out. Going out, even when she did not particularly enjoy being out, became part of her struggle for control and autonomy from a partner who, she felt, treated her like a child, telling her what she could and could not do. All five women described effects on their self-esteem and PE illustrated the way this limited awareness:

> Well I got to the point in the end, I didn't feel no way about anything. And maybe that is why I never noticed what was going on as far as him and R was concerned, that's what I . . . because I wasn't anyway, I wasn't, I had no feelings of myself, about myself. He'd convinced me that I was just nothing, nothing at all, and I believed that in the end . . . I was walking about in a dream, I mean World War 3 could have started outside the front door and I probably wouldn't have even realised it until it was over. But now, my eyes are open and I can see everything about me, I can sort out the good from the bad. (PE)

Two had also developed severe anxiety-related health problems before they had any suspicions that their children had been sexually abused.

For one of the women interviewed (HS), her past experience of abuse as a child was significant. During the early stages of her son's abuse, she had blocked out her own childhood experience and was unable to draw on it to make sense of her concerns: 'There was something drastically wrong. And no one could put their finger on what it was. But sexual interference didn't enter my head.' Two years later, after she had remembered and redefined her own experience as abuse, similar concerns arose again about her son's behaviour, and this time something 'clicked' in her mind. Once the possibility of sexual abuse had occurred to her, she questioned the child and confirmed her suspicion.

Two other women seemed to have had a low level of awareness for reasons other than their own experiences of violence. For CL, her own lack of confidence as a parent was reflected in her perception that her husband got on well with her daughter, since he seemed able to do things she could not with the child. The second (FP) adopted a more detached approach to family life, less concerned with interpreting behaviour than other women, reckoning that family relationships are always difficult to some extent and the best approach is to accept it rather than confront every problem. Hence, though her husband's relationship with his daughter was not particularly close or affectionate, she did not see it as particular cause for concern, since all his children had seemed a nuisance to him. While she had wondered if there was anything wrong with her daughter, the child had 'got uptight' when asked, 'and I'd, rather than quarrel with her, I'd say all right, when you're ready you tell me, you know'. The child later said she did not tell her mother because she thought she was happy in the marriage and did not want to break it up, to which the mother commented that you try not to let children see the problems in your marriage.

It is difficult to assess in retrospect when women may have deflected observations they might have made in response to the threat they posed. However, too much should not be made of 'denial' given the complexity of the interactions surrounding secrecy. CL, who suffered debilitating guilt, had been told that her daughter had been abused by her husband while they were all three in bed together and she was asleep. It is quite likely that she would be seen as denying her own involvement by her claim not to have known. However, it is also possible, given that children being abused commonly freeze and 'play possum' (Summit, 1983) and that her husband penetrated the child's vagina with his fingers, that she was in fact asleep and unaware of what was happening. Sirles and Franke's (1989) study of mothers' responses found that incidents of abuse that occurred when the women were in the house were amongst the most difficult and threatening circumstances and were more likely to be disbelieved for this reason. CL's difficulty in believing the abuse may be attributable partly therefore to the loss and guilt attached to not having known. PE, who expressed the least guilt of all the women about not having known, also expressed a clear recognition of the way in which her partner had manipulated the situation and her perceptions: 'I would say, I mean these men know what they're doing and they're crafty. So you wouldn't sort of see what was going on.'

SUSPECTING

When women do become suspicious that a child of theirs is being sexually abused, why does this not lead to immediate action to protect the child? One answer to this is that suspecting is not the same as knowing, and suspicions can remain unconfirmed for a considerable period of time. Uncertainty of this kind, often alongside continued experiences of violence against themselves, involved intense ambivalence and confusion, and women often fluctuated between trying to find out more to obtain proof and trying to avert further loss by ignoring the evidence that was there. For two women, thinking about this period of their lives was clearly still immensely painful, and they were unable to recall it fully in the interviews. Again the accounts illustrated the complexity of interaction surrounding discovery, with clear information about what was happening often inaccessible, confusion and conflict over the interpretation of what evidence was available, and also over its evaluation, that is, what is normal and what is abuse?

In two cases the child's abuse had been ongoing for two to three years and five years respectively before the mothers began to suspect. In both, the balance of losses and gains attached to discovery changed as the child's and/or mother's resources increased, allowing suspicions to develop. In one the abusive man left the home, reducing the costs to the child of revealing her distress. In the other, the child getting older made her more difficult to control and the mother's increased self-worth and availability enabled her to 'notice things' that seemed wrong.

The ability to confirm suspicions depended not only on the woman's motivation (although that was clearly important) but on the interaction with both her child and the abuser. The option of simply asking children was less realistic for younger children than older, and three of the women had begun to suspect when their children were under 5. One 5-year-old child reacted angrily when asked questions, leaving her mother anxious at whether she was causing her more harm: 'Sometimes with her she would give me the opportunity to ask the right question at the right time but it would still be met with a smack round the face or scream at me' (AN). Two mothers of older children who became suspicious that 'something was going on' between them and their partners also felt awkward about asking direct questions, although a third confronted her daughter directly, but in such rage that it would be unlikely to enable a child to tell. The difficulty of asking questions (as well as eliciting answers) should not be surprising. Parents' reluctance to talk about sex with their children is one of the main reasons that few warn their children effectively of the possibility of sexual abuse (Finkelhor, 1986b). Sex is often a taboo subject between mothers and daughters (Cornwell, 1984), even without the extra difficulty of the mother's own partner being involved. Feelings of anger, rejection, fear and self-doubt compound the difficulties.

Three who confronted partners about their suspicions also met with conflict and confusion. Two who felt their partners' behaviour with their daughters (including jealousy and possessiveness, sharing a bath and encouraging a child to run around naked between the ages of 8 and 12) was wrong were accused of being sick, with sexual hang-ups themselves, and began to believe these accusations. The difficulty of 'drawing the line' between normal father–daughter relationships and abuse, the ambiguity of the evidence available and conflict over its meaning meant women continually experienced self-doubt about their suspicions and often self-blame for having them in the first place. KV described this:

> I thought am I making, it must be me, I'm imagining this, you know, fancy me imagining that about my husband, he's interested in my daughter, what can you say? . . . I'd get these feelings of suspicions and then blame myself, I'd think oh fancy thinking that, that's terrible, that's really, that's real odd thinking that of your husband, you're a bit funny. (KV)

LH appeared to experience no such doubt about the validity of her suspicions, despite denials from both husband and daughter, although her distress at what she witnessed and defined as a love affair meant she continually pushed them to the back of her mind, as described in Chapter 3. However her account illustrates in a different way the difficulty of 'drawing the line' between normal and abusive behaviour since she cited as evidence of the child's abuse past incidents some of which could possibly have a quite innocent meaning. These included her daughter at age 12 once helping her husband to undress and get into bed when he was sick, and at age 13 telling her grandmother that her father sometimes dressed her. The fact that both these incidents now seem indicative of abuse illustrates the way evidence never speaks for itself but is always interpreted through current consciousness and also the different ways the problem may be defined which are examined later in this chapter.

Suspicion is characterised by the inaccessibility of clear information about events conducted in secrecy and uncertainty about the meaning of the information available. One of the problems involved in the discovery of sexual abuse is that even when evidence is obtained it frequently disappears again. There is rarely physical, visible evidence, and hence the construction of reality is precarious. The sense of confusion this generates was illustrated by AN, whose daughter's ambivalence about telling was reflected in dropping hints then refusing to say any more, or drawing pictures then wiping them out. This left her wondering: 'Had I actually heard her say that or did I imagine it? Did she really draw a sausage shape for the reasons I thought she'd drawn it or was it just a sausage shape?' The tendency to rely on visible information in circumstances of such confusion and potential loss meant two women interpreted negative results of medical examinations as indicating no abuse had occurred.

Validation from friends and relatives that they too felt something was wrong was an important part of a cumulative process of discovery, and disbelief could set it back considerably. Indirect validation from knowledge that sexual abuse happened in other families was also important. Ultimately however it was the evidence of those involved, the abuser and the child, that most convincingly confirmed suspicions, and obtaining this could become a preoccupation above all else. PE described an incident when she had spent a night at a friend's, leaving her partner to 'cool down' after violence against herself, and returned to find further evidence:

> I came back early in the morning, which is something I'd never done, and the doors were locked, and when he came down, she, he was undressed and I'd gone straight upstairs, and there was a cup of coffee either side of the bed, and the bed was still warm and everything, and I'd gone running into R's bedroom and pulled the covers back, and she had no clothes on, which my R always slept with clothes on, always, and I said to her, I said what the hell's gone on in here? I know something's gone on. She started screaming and tried to hit me. And he got violent, and in the end, he just walked out, and R got dressed and she went out, and I sat here, and I knew but I didn't know, it was sort of staring me in the face. But *no one would sort of say*, I even threatened R that I would take her to the doctor's, and that, but *she still wouldn't say anything*. (emphasis added) (PE)

Women were often ambivalent about confirming their suspicions, wanting but not wanting to know and their motivation to overcome the resistance of others to open awareness therefore fluctuated. They were also often faced with multiple, conflicting and changing versions of events and their meaning, from the child, the abuser and others who became involved. The centrality of the family in women's construction of reality, their sense of their role as mediators, combined in some cases with a lack of psychological separation, meant that achieving a version of events agreed by all family members was often a central preoccupation once information suggesting abuse was acquired. As well as the ongoing inaccessibility of information, the interpretation of evidence involved assessment, in relation to the women's former knowledge of the actors and of the period in which abuse had taken place, to achieve a fit. This process, involving reinterpreting past incidents and assessing new information to construct a revised version of the period of abuse, was referred to by several women as 'piecing the jigsaw together', and could take a considerable period of time.

There was often strong resistance from both the abuser and the child to the mother confirming suspicions. Two women obtained irrefutable evidence unwittingly, one 'catching him' and the other finding the child with semen on her hair and clothes when she had been in the care of her 17-year-old brother. Others however had to make persistent attempts to obtain further evidence and to resolve the conflict between the accounts of those involved. Six women felt that they had placed their children under considerable pressure and three of these had threatened the child themselves to make them say what had happened and who was the abuser. One had also pretended to the child that she already knew from the abusive man in order to persuade her to tell. All these obtained the information they needed from the child (although not necessarily the full details).

Three women had never obtained their children's word although they had all asked. For all of them this was a major sticking point in their process of discovery. Two seemed to have asked only once and their ambivalence about finding out, and confusion about the information they had, prevented their successfully overcoming the child's fear and ambivalence. The third asked with such anger that it would be unlikely to encourage a child to 'confess'. Although her daughter had implicitly told her in many ways, including asking her mother to leave the home, she had never 'admitted' the relationship with her father.

Only three of the children in this sample told voluntarily, all when the abuser had left or was not a member of the household (although one was a temporary absence). The threats commonly made to children by abusers and the complex feelings of fear, guilt and responsibility the abuse and secrecy engender mean that children are more likely to tell the further away the abuser is. This is one of the reasons that concerns about sexual abuse sometimes arise for the first time during custody disputes.

For all fourteen women, the word of the child was particularly important in confirming suspicions, whether by its presence or its absence. All those living with the abusive man had however also confronted him to obtain his account as well. Of these eight, three of the men had admitted the abuse and five persistently denied it to the mother. The three whose husbands had admitted the abuse, and who also had obtained the word of the child, were those women who had most successfully resolved the process of discovery, both resolving conflict between the versions of those involved and achieving a fit between the new knowledge and their previous versions of the past. Of these three men, however, only one was consistent about admitting the abuse, the other two continued to deny it to others and one had reverted to denying it to the woman, sending her letters from prison accusing her of lying which caused her considerable distress. In these cases, breaking through the abuser's denial was not a once and for all point. Rather, confession seems to have been a part of the process of manipulation, strategic when it seemed impossible to avoid the secret coming out and yet possible to achieve a resolution within the family.

The effects of denial from abusive men on women's ability to confirm their suspicions are illustrated by PE's account of attempting to resolve conflicting accounts:

> I wanted to believe R and I wanted to believe him. I wanted to believe that they were both telling the truth, but I knew that one of them had to be lying. And in one way I wanted it to be R that was lying to me, obviously. (PE)

In this context, a sense of having confirmed suspicions was often followed by recurring doubts, the inconsistency of evidence making reality precarious.

Of the five women faced with persistent denial, four had since separated from the abusive men although two of these not by their own choice. The two who had chosen to leave had more or less confirmed their suspicions despite the abuser's denial, although both had some ongoing unresolved issues. The three who had either stayed with a denying abuser or not chosen to separate had all been unable fully to resolve their discovery. None of their responses are properly described as denial or disbelief. Two in fact did believe the abuse had taken place, and the third remained uncertain what to believe. The latter's account (CL) will be described in some detail later in this chapter to illustrate the process of becoming stuck in a state of unconfirmed suspicion.

Even achieving verbal acknowledgement from both parties is not the end of the story. For most women there was a continuing process of interpreting new information and reassessing the past to reconcile the two, 'piecing the jigsaw together'. Only four of the women had less than a year to reassess, six had three years and one had seven years in which the abuse had taken place in secret. Even those women who described 'instant belief' also illustrated the process of reassessment and the importance of piecing together events in their accounts. Past knowledge of the child's behaviour problems, of the abusive man's propensity to violence, the child's age and access to other sources of knowledge about sex, awareness of the reasons children find telling about sexual abuse difficult and information from friends and public sources about sexual abuse in general all contributed to this process of interpretation.

Given the losses involved in discovery and the resistance of those involved, to resolve the process of discovery successfully and sustain belief takes considerable persistence on the mother's behalf. A sense that the situation can be improved if accepted is vital and the loss of hope that anything but further loss is possibly a major contributing factor to the failure to confirm suspicions. A number of factors were identifiable as gains, which could therefore give a 'reason to believe'. For one woman, the difficulty of living with uncertainty made confirmation in part a relief. For two, the discovery that their husbands, who had consistently criticised everything they did, had now done something clearly wrong themselves also gave some relief. As EJ put it, despite her horror and panic, 'I thought I've really got something on him now'. For another, her ambivalence over belief was resolved when she realised that the fear, worry and tension her husband caused her meant she could not live with him any more anyway. The desire to recover the child's trust and to restore their own sense of being good mothers could also provide a reason to believe.

Not all the women in this study had successfully confirmed their suspicions. Only one of these (CL) would conventionally be categorised as disbelieving or denying the abuse, but to examine her account in some detail suggests the inadequacy of these concepts. CL had come home from work one day to be told by a relative living with her that her mother (the child's grandmother) had taken her daughter (aged 5) down to the police station because she had been sexually abused. Her husband had already been arrested at his workplace and her father also came by and told her. Her sister had told the school that D was 'getting sore' and had apparently been interfered with by a man in the household. The school had contacted the police, the police told social workers, and the social workers got the grandmother to take D to the station. No one had apparently attempted to contact CL. When she found out on her return from work, she went to the police station and was refused any information. The social worker did not visit her until two weeks later.

The emotional impact of this discovery was still very immediate three years later and she talked in the interview as if it had happened yesterday. She said repeatedly 'I was the last to know' and 'They wouldn't give me no information', expressing a continuing sense of loss, isolation and rejection. She was clear that she had not minded the police being involved if her husband had committed a crime and her distress was on her own behalf not in defence of him:

> It's 'cos I think I wasn't involved, told or involved in anything what was happening, I think that's what was the worst part about it. Nobody even came up and said well we've charged your husband with this or with that

or whatever the case may be, nobody told me nothing. As I say I even went down the station and nobody even gave me any information. *It felt that I was an outsider. Instead of being a next of kin of both of them, I was the one that was told nothing.* Everybody else knew except me. As I say, my brother-in-law knew more, my parents knew more. I was the last one. Where I thought I should have been the first, or been informed, I wasn't. I think that's what even made it, made me feel worse, because I wasn't informed by anybody. (emphasis added) (CL)

It may be that this experience resonates with her past sense of isolation and rejection by her family, but the passage underlined also indicates the loss involved in relation to women's identification with family and their role as mediators, both between family members and between family and public agencies. Given the loss the discovery of sexual abuse itself involves, the handling of disclosure to exclude mothers in this way runs the risk of seriously exacerbating it and increasing their vulnerability to pressure from the abuser.

The sense of being excluded continued for CL throughout the intervention process, in which she felt that everyone was against her, that she had no part in decisions and that she was herself blamed for the abuse, in particular by the suggestion that if she and her husband had had a better sexual relationship it would not have happened. In this context, where so much guilt was attached to the occurrence of abuse and the intervention process felt only like pressure, there was little if anything to be gained by believing the abuse had happened. She seemed to have had no sense of any possible positive outcome: 'See, I had nothing or anything on my side . . . in a sense I had no chance, there's nothing I could have done . . . I felt like I was hitting a dead end when it hit me.'

In addition, her inability to confirm the ongoing suspicions and doubts she was left with revolved around her husband's persistent denial and the fact that her child had never told her. For all the women in this study the accounts of the child and/or the abuser (where a member of the household) were particularly important and the word of others carried considerably less weight. CL had confronted her husband early on, feeling confused and angry, not sure what she thought had happened at this point but angry that everyone else seemed to know and she did not know what was going on. He denied it, leaving her more confused. 'I just didn't know what to believe, and he just kept on saying he didn't do it.'

Three years later he still denied it to her, despite having pleaded guilty in court on the advice of his barrister to help the child (and, of course, lessen the sentence). He did not deny that the child had been abused but suggested that her brother, who was also living with them, was responsible.

Her account illustrates the importance of not seeing parents' denial as a unitary phenomenon, since, where they have different access to information about abuse, the doubts of one may be the result of a persistent campaign by the other:

> I didn't think he'd do a thing like that . . . he said so much that he didn't do it, that I didn't actually think he did do it because he convinced me so much in his own way that he didn't do it. He said that he wanted to prove to me that he didn't do it but there's no way he could. So I was sort of, a bit doubtful 'cos I had all them saying that he did do it, you know. (CL)

When asked what she thought now, whether he had done it or not, she replied: 'Well I still got that little bit of doubt in the back of my mind, but he still, he still says he didn't and for him to say that, it makes me wonder.' Her confusion did not indicate agreement with the abuse. It indicated rather a failure of power to overcome her husband's denial.

CL had also asked her daughter, although she had been uncertain whether to do so or not in case she upset her. She did do so a couple of days after the initial discovery but this did not help to resolve her confusion: 'When I asked her she said no to me, that's why I couldn't understand what was going on.' This continued to be a major sticking point:

> You see, if D had actually come up and said mummy, daddy did do it, or something like that, I might have felt different, but no one's really, D's not really come up and I think she's the one that would know more than anybody who done it. (CL)

She had not talked much more to the child about it, having been advised by the guardian ad litem to let her forget and also finding the subject difficult. She had gathered 'bits and pieces' of information from the social worker who visited her and from what she heard in court, but these sources of evidence did not carry enough weight to overturn so much of her past reality. Hence she still felt 'I had nothing to go on, only by what everybody else was saying to me'. She remained stuck in self-doubt, not having developed a way to mediate successfully between the conflicting versions of events.

She had also been unable to fit the bits of information she obtained into her pre-existing version of the past. She had been told that the child had been abused while in bed with her and her husband:

> This is why I find it hard, because if it had happened I might have noticed it, or felt something happening in a sense, I would have sensed it. But this is it, I didn't sense nothing or feel nothing, that's why I find it so hard to believe, 'cos I was supposed to have been there, in a sense. (CL)

This is neither a blanket denial nor a self-justifying account. She added that it was made harder to believe by the fact that she was a light sleeper. Had she been justifying her ignorance or denying her knowledge, she would be more likely to have described herself as a heavy sleeper. It is rather an indication of the extent of the loss belief would carry in such circumstances.

There were three other cases in this sample in which the failure to confirm suspicions and to establish open communication, at least with the child, was marked. All believed the abuse had taken place, but either the refusal of the child to talk about it or their own sense of loss inhibited further moves towards open awareness. Other women too, who had re-solved the process enough to choose to separate from abusive partners in response, still had some unresolved areas as a result of their own and/or the child's continued ambivalence about communicating. EJ had left her hus-band over ten years ago, her abused daughter was now an adult and they had a close relationship which meant that her daughter phoned her for support when she had recurring nightmares about her father's abuse. How-ever, EJ still did not know the full details of what had happened: 'I think she couldn't bring herself to tell me in any detail. And I suppose I chickened out, and I didn't want to hear, if I'm honest.' This daughter had also suggested that perhaps her sisters had been abused as well. EJ did not think so, 'but is it that I don't want to think so? I don't know'. Once there was no further risk to the children and no action to be taken, there seemed little to be gained by pursuing the information further.

There are dangers to such unresolved areas since women may feel unable to come to terms with events they do not fully know about, and/or their lives may be disrupted again when further information is volunteered at a later date. RD described her frustration at her daughter's refusal to talk about her abuse, and the limits this set to her knowledge: 'Sometimes I want to catch her and shake her, for her to tell me. But it wouldn't be the right way. I think she'll tell me when she's ready.'

KNOWING

Full knowledge of the events is not the end of the discovery process. Events must also be ascribed meaning and this meaning may change over time, influenced by later family interactions, public response and information as well as the mother's own experience. The process of discovery involves defining what is acceptable and what is abuse within a continuum of behaviour and relationships, that is, 'where to draw the line'. Furthermore, 'abuse' is not a monolithic category but involves evaluation of degrees of seriousness. Such evaluation of the seriousness of child sexual abuse is by

no means uniform amongst professionals. One survey of professional attitudes however found the type of sexual activity an important influence,
intercourse being seen as more serious than handling (Eisenberg *et al.*,
1987).

There is no agreed definition of what exactly constitutes child sexual
abuse.[1] A broad agreement exists amongst professionals however that
essentially it involves the exploitation of a power relationship over children
for the sexual gratification of an adult or significantly older child.[2] One
definition states that this pertains:

> whether or not this activity involves explicit coercion by any means,
> whether or not it involves genital or physical contact, whether or not
> initiated by the child, and whether or not there is discernible harmful
> outcome in the short term.
>
> (SCOSAC, 1984, cited in Glaser and Frosh, 1988, p. 5)

The crucial defining factor is the power relationship, and the inability of
children to give informed consent. Any involvement of children in sexual
activities in this context therefore involves a betrayal of the trust their
vulnerability requires them to place in those with greater knowledge,
capabilities and access to resources.

Such a definition is not uniformly accepted and conflict continues over
specific acts. There is currently a tendency to exclude acts in which no
physical contact is involved, such as flashing, showing pornography or
voyeurism (Cooper and Ball, 1987; La Fontaine, 1990). This is problematic
in the light of evidence that, even for adult women, flashing is both
violating in itself and relies in part for its impact on the threat of further
assault (Kelly, 1988a). Moreover, persistent flashing by a father, for instance, carries a different threat from a single incident by a stranger. To
incorporate the experience of children, definitions must take account not
only of the acts involved, but their persistence over time and the relationship and access the abuser has to the child.

As Kelly (1988c) has argued, conflicts over definition reflect the context
of male dominance, in which it is in men's interests as a group and as the
main perpetrators of sexual violence to ensure that the definitions of sexual
violence are as limited as possible. For women and girls to define their own
experience as abuse is a difficult and complex process, because of the
myths and stereotypes which surround sexual violence, the coping strategies they adopt of forgetting and minimising, and the need to challenge
dominant definitions. The difficulties for mothers in defining their child's
experience as abuse reflect the further complexity of women's contradictory position as mothers. While they are in a position of power to define
their child's experience and often have to do so on the basis of limited

evidence, their difficulties in doing so reflect their position as women for whom dominant definitions require that sexual violence is minimised and further their frequent sense of powerlessness as mothers. Women who were able clearly to define their own experiences as sexual violence (including everyday harassment, the use of pornography by partners as well as child-hood experiences) and who had a sense of their own power as adults were clearer in defining their child's abuse and understanding its implications.

For several women the term 'sexual abuse' had been imposed on their child's experience by others and its meaning was vague. 'Abuse' is by definition wrong and those who had a clear definition tended to talk in terms of right and wrong behaviour (i.e. the transgression of moral rules) and to recognise the issues of power involved. However, not all of those who saw the abuse as clearly wrong recognised its implications for the child. Two questions merit consideration therefore: first, what factors inhibited the definition of the behaviour concerned as wrong; and, second, for what other reasons was it defined as wrong other than the abuse of power involved?

For several women their own subjective sense of powerlessness was reflected in lack of recognition of the power of adults and vulnerability of children and consequent confusion over the implications of abuse. The age of the abuser could also influence the definition of abuse, abuse by teenage boys being seen as 'not as bad' as that by adult men by virtue of their lesser power and responsibility for their own actions. The apparent intentions of the abuser were also significant. Thus, one woman had accepted her hus-band's definition of his behaviour as sex education and still accepted his insistence that he had not intended harm. The justification of abusive behaviour as sex education to children is a common part of the victimi-sation process (Berliner and Conte, 1990). Perceptions of the abuser's intention to harm are also significant influences on women's definitions of themselves as battered (Sedlak, 1988; Bograd, 1988b) and on professional definitions of parental behaviour as physical abuse (Herzberger and Tennen, 1988).

The effects on the child were a further source of clarity or confusion. One woman's child had told her by saying her father did things she did not like. This enabled her to confront him with clarity that it was wrong to be doing anything the child did not like. Another interpreted her daughter's refusal to tell her as 'because she liked it'. A third (BM) expressed ongoing confusion about the relationship between 'abuse' and pleasure and/or harm, reflected in her instructions to her husband to do nothing the children did not like and exacerbated by the fact that similar activities had affected two children quite differently, one reacting with obvious and long-term distress (although not evident until some time after the abuse had stopped) and the other seeming apparently unaffected. The age of the child was also referred to as a defining factor in abuse and it is likely that the older the child the less the significance of the power relationship is evident. Finkelhor's study of a random sample of families in Boston which explored lay definitions of abuse found whether the child resisted or not to be a significant factor influencing definition, along with the age of child and abuser and the nature of the act (Finkelhor and Redfield, 1984).

The relationship context of the abuse also influenced definition of behaviour, which was complicated not only by the context of male dominance but by the privacy of family life and the secrecy surrounding much of the abuse. Women thus had little information on what happens in other families and often limited evidence on what was happening in their own. The confusion some expressed about what is normal sexual behaviour between fathers and daughters was a real difficulty, illustrating Johnson's argument that such relationships involve a continuum in which seductiveness and manipulation are common and incest the extreme end (Johnson, 1982). Different rules are often applied to behaviour in family relationships than to behaviour by those outside and one woman defined her husband's abuse of a visiting child more clearly as abuse partly because of the lack of an ongoing relationship within which, if things went wrong, you could make up for them later. The emotional context of the relationship also influences women's definitions of themselves as battered (Sedlak, 1988). For this reason, mothers' definitions may not necessarily be in accord with the common perception thought to exist that abuse by a biological father is more serious than abuse by anyone else (La Fontaine, 1990).

One commonly used definition of 'sexual abuse' which attempts to come closer to specific behaviour than that given above refers to activities which 'violate the social taboos of family roles' (DoH, 1991a). This however implies both knowledge of and consensus about such taboos which may not exist. The account of one woman suggested widespread support amongst a middle-class parents' support group for practices such as breast-feeding children during, or having children witness, their parents having sex, which many professionals would consider abusive or at least borderline.

Further sources of confusion were similar to those expressed in academic and public debate. One woman had read of practices in other cultures which were not regarded there as abusive (such as stroking male babies' genitals to calm them in Japan) and questioned the definition of her children's abuse on this basis. She also expressed the common concern about where 'good touch' becomes 'bad touch'. Having wanted her husband to become closer to her children and include physical intimacy in that, she was still confused about differentiating what was positive and negative in his response.

Only one mother (BM) in this study knew about her husband's abuse of their children (touching their genitals) while it was going on, over a period of years. For her too, there was a process of discovery, since, although she knew of the events and had sometimes been present, she was uncertain about their meaning and did not see them as abusive at the time. The distinctive factor about the incident which prompted her concern was that her daughter (aged 11) had complained. BM stopped her husband touching any of the children after this, but explained her failure to do so earlier, 'I didn't know what sexual abuse was, you see', and previously had instructed him only not to do anything the children would not like. She still however (eight years later) expressed considerable confusion about what abuse was.

Many of the sources of her confusion have been discussed above – the indirect relationship between abuse, visible effects and pleasure/harm, a sense of powerlessness which obscured the power relationship between adults and children, exacerbated in her case by a child-rearing style that deliberately minimised the guidance role of parents in the interests of children defining their own needs. However, her own background seemed also to contribute to inability to recognise abuse, through the confusion she expressed about sex, intimacy and violence, which seemed all rolled together for her. She expressed continuing conflict about her own childhood, initially describing it as happy but later talking of her separation from her parents as the type of abuse she suffered. She had had little experience of family life herself, and little experience of any form of intimacy prior to her marriage. She had been single until she was 29 and talked of marrying largely as an attempt to resolve her anxieties about sexuality and gain social acceptability. She said that her sex education had started with her marriage, and from the beginning sex and violence were intertwined. Her husband had proposed to her saying that he was afraid he would rape her if they did not marry quickly. This conflation continued since she talked of his friendship with another woman later in terms of whether he 'would assault her', meaning whether it would become a sexual relationship. Marriage seemed equated with sex for her, since, when asked questions about her experience of marriage, she replied almost entirely in terms of sex. She was consequently engaged in a battle for control with her husband in which she talked of 'making him wait' for sex, while at the same time regarding it as part of her role to contain his sexual 'needs' within the marriage.

Her marriage was characterised by similar struggles and conflict over most areas, in particular child-rearing about which both her husband and his mother had claimed to know a great deal more than her. She had not in fact accepted her husband's definitions of his actions as sex education uncritically but her attempt to challenge them was ineffectual, given her own confusion over what was right and wrong in child-rearing. Her account of this was charged both with this history of conflict, and with her desire to give her children what she had never had herself, intimacy and physical closeness with their parents. Her own experience of intimacy having been restricted to sex seemed to inhibit her from considering alternative ways of achieving this.

> I wasn't quite sure what sexual abuse was, you see, I mean if it was, my mother-in-law thought it was wrong to kiss babies, and it was wrong to cuddle them after they were 6 months old, and it was wrong to . . . you know, what was right? I was a bit confused about what was right and how to instruct my husband as to how to treat them, you see . . . he said oh children have their sexuality and they . . . I said it was wrong to arouse it, and he said well why is it wrong, you know. I mean he was just about as ignorant as me as to, what was, what was right, I suppose incest is obviously wrong but I didn't know exactly where to tell him to stop . . . where to draw the line with the touching, you see. (BM)

Even when full information about events is available, a rare occurrence in cases of incestuous abuse, the difficulty of defining what is normal and what is abuse recurs.

BM's account comes nearest of all the women in this sample to the common perception of a mother colluding with the abuse of her children, since she knew about it and made no attempt initially to protect her children from her husband. However the concept of collusion does not adequately encompass either the changes in her perception over time or the constant and continuing conflict with her husband over the meaning of his behaviour. Her husband had continued to define what he had done as being 'too loving', a definition which she disputed, and her own process of redefining these incidents, in response either to her daughter's behaviour or to outside information, had involved a continual and ineffective struggle with him, in which she seemed locked, still trying to change his understanding of what he had done. Her attempts to achieve a shared definition of reality were similar to those which other women made over conflicting versions of events, and reflected both her own definition of her role as mediator between her children and husband (which she performed reluctantly) and the moral significance she attached to husband and wife as a 'united front'. As in the case of CL described earlier, her failure to mediate successfully was a failure of power in relation to her husband, this time to counter his definition of his behaviour effectively.

This section has illustrated the factors that may inhibit the definition of abusive behaviour as wrong. However, defining it as wrong does not necessarily reflect a recognition of the abuse of power involved. Three women reacted with horror and anger to the abuse but yet had little sense of their own power as adults or their children's vulnerability, speaking of them as equal in capabilities. One of these blamed her daughter as 'the seducer'. The other two expressed little empathy for their children, and one of the children had been taken permanently into care. For these women, the problem was defined primarily as sex rather than power. Their own lack of any control over their sexuality (one had been raped consistently by her husband, another 'knew you couldn't say no' and the third expressed guilt that she did not 'have sex often enough') was reflected in fear and hatred of sex. The abuse was therefore particularly threatening to them, reflected in anger at the abusive men being 'perverts/nonces'. In this context, anger at the abuser does not necessarily indicate empathy for the child.[3]

These issues suggest that it is not enough to offer women evidence of specific activities on which to define their children's experience as abuse, since their own feelings of powerlessness and lack of control over sexuality may inhibit their ability to understand the meaning and implications for the child.

SUMMARY AND CONCLUSIONS

The answers to the question 'did the mother know?' are likely to be far from simple. There are multiple possible combinations of awareness where a child is being sexually abused in the family, and it cannot be concluded that because a child thinks the mother knows she does or because a child thinks the mother does not know that she does not. The question of knowing itself is over-simplistic since it is possible to know of events without understanding their meaning, to be confused over the boundaries between normal and abusive behaviour but open to help which clarifies definition. For most women, with much less direct access to information about events, there are further issues of the interpretation of evidence which often has no obvious direct relationship to abusive events. Evidence which seems an indicator of abuse to professionals may well seem open to a number of other interpretations to the mother.

The process which workers go through when discovering or recognising the sexual abuse of a child is in many ways similar. Recognition is rarely straightforward. Evidence is often inaccessible and open to varying inter-pretation and evaluation. Despite the language of diagnosis sometimes used, sexual abuse is not a disease with clearly identifiable characteristics, but an interaction between individuals. Discovery is the product of further interactions, between social workers and other professionals, and between professionals, different members of the family and others. Reality is con-structed through this interaction and the complexity of communication surrounding child sexual abuse means it is often precarious and uncertain, for workers as well as for mothers. In my study, social workers showed a reluctance to accept evidence reported by others (including some very clear medical evidence) on its own, preferring communication with those most directly involved. They were also sometimes anxious about asking questions on such a 'delicate subject' and unable to elicit the information they needed or resolve conflicting accounts when they did. Once they identified abuse, social workers, like mothers, recognised evidence that they had missed in the past (Hooper, 1990).

The analysis of mothers' discovery process presented in this chapter suggests that assessments which attempt to categorise mothers' responses around simple dichotomies – knowing or not knowing, believing or disbelieving – are inappropriate. Rather, there are a number of ways in which workers may contribute to women's ability to believe that a child has been sexually abused. Both dimensions to the discovery process – the availability, interpretation and evaluation of evidence on the one hand, and the losses and gains involved in changing awareness on the other – need to be considered throughout. Work may need to focus on increasing the availability of information, for example working with the child to enable her to tell the mother, helping her to write a story that can be shown to the mother or using an existing statement if there is one. It may also need to address the interpretation of evidence, for example helping women to understand their children's silence or denial. Children's reluctance to tell of abuse should not be attributed to fault in the mother – to attribute it to the mother's unavailability or a poor relationship generally is to underestimate the difficulties of telling inherent in the experience of child sexual abuse and the complexity of the discovery process. General information – that false allegations from children are rare, for example – is useful. Equally important however is interpreting the behaviour of the individual child (and possibly of the man who perpetrated the abuse) in order to achieve a revised version of the past which makes sense in the light of new information.

A third level involves the evaluation of evidence, that is, the definition of abuse. This should not be assumed to be self-evident. There is room for confusion in a number of areas: the relationship between pleasure and harm if the child appeared to enjoy the sexual contact, the significance of the power relationship between adults and children in defining abuse, the indirect relationship between harm and visible effects. Women are more likely to be able to define their child's experience as abuse if they have a sense of their own power as adults and of a right to control over their own sexuality.

Throughout, the balance of losses and gains needs to be borne in mind. If awareness involves only further losses, addressing belief via the availability, interpretation and evaluation of evidence may not be success-ful, but may instead trigger coping strategies which redefine the available evidence. Stressing the devastating effects of disbelief on the child may well be counterproductive, for example, if the mother has already dis-believed her. Indicating the positive effects the mother's belief and support can still have is likely to be more helpful. The association of femininity (and especially motherhood) with selflessness appears to make some workers dismissive of the need women have for hope that things can improve in order to give them a 'reason to believe'.

5 Working it out
The context and process of response

When the sexual abuse of a child is discovered by professionals, it is a common requirement that the abuser and the child should be separated. Mothers are therefore commonly faced with a choice between their partner (if he is the known or suspected abuser) or another resident family member (e.g. son) on the one hand and the abused child on the other. If they are unwilling to exclude the former from the household, the abused child is likely to be received into care. Whether temporary or permanent separation from the abuser is expected depends on the treatment available for abusers and the degree of optimism about its effectiveness. In general the less the possibility of rehabilitating abusers with the rest of the family (if all wish this) is considered, the greater the expectations of mothers to make a long-term choice between abuser and child.

In this study, the women's discovery and hence their process of response had in most cases preceded the involvement of agencies. Women did not necessarily start from the premise that a choice between the abuser and the child was necessary and several attempted, with varying degrees of success, both to keep the family together and to prevent the abuse recurring. Neither did they always assume that the abuse should be reported to agencies. It is sometimes assumed that women who do not separate immediately from an abusive partner (Faller, 1988a) or who do not report to agencies (Wilk and McCarthy, 1986) are thereby colluding with the abuse. This implies there is only one correct course of action to take on the discovery of sexual abuse in the family and ignores both the complexity of the situation and the risk-taking nature of child-rearing in general. As Freeman argues, in many situations there are 'a band of possible reasonable decisions' in child-rearing (1983, p. 245) and the discovery of child sexual abuse is no exception. Women whose children are sexually abused face a similar task to professionals who must both assess the risk to the child of further abuse and take some risks since predictions based on such assessments can never be 100 per cent certain. Mothers of course have less information on which to base their judgements and considerably more to lose. This chapter aims to describe the women's responses within their context, identifying factors which influenced them, and to elaborate the process of response.

There was a strong sense in which the concept of choice was of limited relevance, given the structural constraints on women's options, the losses the discovery of sexual abuse entailed and their own struggles for survival. Choices are always made within a social, economic and political context and hence raise questions about how that context is constructed. The social context in which child care is by and large women's private business, economic dependence on men the structure expected to support this and lone parenting penalised socially and economically (Millar, 1987) is one which constrains women's choices and perpetuates disadvantage for those who separate from abusive partners. To choose 'for the child' means women are likely to exchange economic dependence on men for dependence on state benefits and low-paid work (Joshi, 1987) or alternatively to replace dependence on one man with dependence on another. The low levels of public day care in Britain (Cohen, 1990) and its stigmatised nature increase the degree of responsibility women must take on if they 'choose' to parent alone. Furthermore, their ability to protect children from further contact with abusive men is limited by the common failures of the legal system to back the efforts they make.

Economics, social policy and the law all reflect and are reinforced by dominant ideologies concerning marriage, motherhood and family. By and large these structures act to constrain mothers from protecting children from violent men rather than to facilitate such action. However, since people act purposefully within structures (Giddens, 1979), there are variations of response. The sources of these are the focus of the first section of this chapter.

Women's responses are influenced by personal as well as public constraints. Their difficulties in making a decision in such a situation of moral conflict reflect not only the social and economic costs involved but the effects of male dominance on women's psychological development. Women faced with the sexual abuse of a child by a partner are sometimes immobilised, unable to make a choice (Myer, 1984; Gomes-Schwartz *et al.*, 1990). The second section examines three broad approaches taken to the problem of choice, reflected in the way women talked about themselves and others, drawing on Gilligan's (1982) analysis of concepts of self and morality. Immobility is located within a survival-orientated response in which the women's own needs were too overwhelming for choice to be meaningful.

While the contexts of women's choices involve both public and personal constraints, the process is considerably more complex than the concept of a choice between separate individuals suggests. Women in this study talked in terms of conflicting relationships and responsibilities and were concerned with a network of interconnected relationships far wider than the abuser and the abused child, extending over time. Where a decision was made which implied choice (to separate from an abusive partner, for instance) it was not one focused around a single event or point in time but one made in the context of both a history and an anticipated future of relationships. Much of the process of response however was less explicit and conscious than this. It was better understood as part of the ongoing processes of negotiating conflicting relationships and mediating between different family members and between family and public agencies, which are as much a part of the role women play as primary carers as is the direct provision of care for dependent children (Graham, 1985). Within this process, changing circumstances led to changing judgements and actions. The conflicts in family networks which child sexual abuse, especially but not only by partners, raised meant women took risks with the child's safety in attempting to resolve them. Ultimately, the relationships involved were often not reconcilable. Nevertheless the attempt to reconcile them represents an extension of women's role as mothers. The third section of this chapter elaborates the process of response and identifies the factors which influenced it.

THE CONTEXT OF RESPONSE: SOCIAL AND ECONOMIC FACTORS

The social context of response bears some similarities to other family decisions. Studies examining the decision to care for an elderly relative note that carers are often unable to talk in terms of a conscious decision, either because there would have been serious problems of conscience and perceived public disapproval had they not cared (Marsden and Abrams, 1987) or because caring for one's own mother was regarded as 'natural' (Lewis and Meredith, 1988). One study noted the even greater social pressure where caring for a spouse is concerned, given the ideology of marriage as the supreme caring relationship, 'in sickness and in health', to the extent that other options were largely excluded and it was not possible to discuss a choice (Ungerson, 1987).

Maternal love, or at least protection, was certainly regarded as 'natural' by all the women interviewed, although this did not preclude conflict. The one woman who had ended up hating her daughter bitterly spoke of herself as unnatural: 'I hate her, I literally hate her and she's my own flesh and blood, there's not many mothers can say they hate their kids but I hate her, I do' (LH). Two others who anticipated or had experienced conflict between a long-term commitment to the abused child and remarriage expressed their ambivalence about the costs the child might impose on their own lives only indirectly or with great difficulty.

There are differences from as well as similarities with the decision to care – first, a direct choice between two family members is involved, which therefore entails conflicting imperatives between mothering and marriage (where a partner is the abuser). In this context, it seemed more possible to talk of decision making in relation to marriage (where more, if still limited, options are open) than to do so in relation to the child. Second, it is even less acceptable to consider alternative options for a child's care than for that of an elderly relative. The emphasis on the primacy of the mother–child bond for child development means that the mother is held directly responsible for the child's welfare, whoever has actually abused the child. Several respondents had relied on temporary alternative sources of care for the child while attempting to resolve the situation, but the consideration of long-term alternatives was not discussed as an option, only as a possible outcome of failure.

This section focuses primarily on those cases where the abuser was a member of the household at the time of the abuse, including those of the two mothers who had separated before they discovered it. While the context of choice is particularly problematic when a partner is the abuser, involving the material and ideological constraints associated with marriage/men, this may not in fact be the most difficult circumstance for mothers. The woman whose son abused her daughter had not overcome her horror at having to choose between them, and it is possible that the conflicts involved in this situation are in some ways worse. While there are not the constraints imposed by economic dependence, neither is there the ideological plus available of being a 'good mother' by excluding the abuser.

Men and mothering

Despite women's increased participation in paid employment, marriage and mothering – 'having a family' – remain the main career for most women. They are combined, however, in various ways, with different implications for response to the sexual abuse of a child by a partner. Graham (1977) has distinguished between women for whom motherhood is central to their life plan and marriage the institutional framework for it and women who reverse the order and for whom child-bearing is the consequence of rather than the reason for marriage. Despite the recent increase in cohabitation and lone mothering, the broad distinction was useful in understanding the varying significance of conflicting relationships. Those women for whom children were the consequence of marriage (or relationships with men) were more likely to attempt to hold on to those relationships despite the sexual abuse and to feel resentment to the child if they could not do so. The degree to which women themselves victimised by their partners become 'entrapped' has also been related to the value accorded marriage (Strube, 1988). Psychological entrapment refers to a decision-making process whereby individuals escalate their commitment to a previously chosen, though failing, course of action, in order to justify previous investments.

It was not possible to separate two groups clearly by their priority to men or mothering, partly because life plans had changed over time. For one woman the sexual abuse itself had provoked a change in priorities. Chronological order also did not necessarily indicate priority. Six of the fifteen women had had children before they married. However, for three of these mothering had been a way of achieving adult status and independence from their families of origin, and marriage, though later, was equally important. In each case the first child became the reason for marriage (for economic support and 'normal family' status), and further children also the consequence.

Moreover, children were not simply the consequence of marriage but in several cases were almost the cost, in that they were expected to be women's contribution to the marital bargain (to bear and care for children in exchange for economic support), to the extent of self-sacrifice where necessary. For one woman whether she could provide children had been an issue from the first mention of marriage, after meeting her partner two or three times. For several others there was an element of self-sacrifice in providing children for the marriage, to the extent of bearing another child despite strong medical advice against it. In this context one woman described feelings of betrayal and rivalry when her husband 'took over' the child from birth (many years before he sexually abused her), since she had 'done this thing for him' (EJ).

While some women expected themselves to provide children as proof of their commitment to the marriage – to the extent that, for one, children seemed fairly interchangeable and she talked of the temptation to snatch a child from someone else when hers was taken into care – for others their attempts to control their own fertility were a site of marital conflict. Control over reproduction was discussed in Chapter 3 as a site of marital conflict. It seems likely to have implications for the way in which women respond to a partner's abuse of a child if they were pressured or forced by him into having the child in the first place. Unplanned conceptions have been found to increase the likelihood of mothers abusing or neglecting children themselves, although these were attributed only to problems in using contraception (Zuravin, 1987). There is some evidence that women who have been sexually abused themselves as children are at particularly high risk of teenage pregnancy, and not only through the direct consequences of forced sexual intercourse (Gershenson *et al.*, 1989). The lack of self-esteem and sense of powerlessness that are often consequences of sexual abuse may lead both to vulnerability to further coercive sexual experiences, and to self-neglect and consequently high levels of risk-taking in contraceptive behaviour.

Ideas of duty in marriage, which appeared to be linked both to class and religious beliefs, were also significant. Three women referred to the duty to make marriage for life, for better or worse. Two of these had in the end separated but one had had four years of suspicion before confirming the abuse and deciding to leave, and one stayed for a year before separating. The third had stayed with her husband and still saw this as a choice, based however on the view that 'I've undertaken to be his wife for life, that's what marriage is . . . if one marries thinking that marriage is only working if it is producing happiness, then no wonder marriage doesn't work for so many people' (BM). This view of marriage and the stigma attached to divorce was expressed by all the middle-class women in the sample (including those whose husbands were not the abusers but with whom there were other problems) and by one of the working-class women (for religious reasons). The working-class women described their marriages more explicitly in terms of a bargain, in which husband's unemployment, drink problems, failure to provide for them and the children financially all reduced the worth of the marriage to them.

The dominant familial ideology was reflected in recurring references by many of the women to the desire to be a 'normal family', that is, with both partner and child(ren). As CL, who was unwilling to choose between her husband and child, said, 'Well I wanted the four of us, 'cos that's what I wanted more than anything, just like a normal family'. One striking difference however was that neither of the two Afro-Caribbean women who participated in the study used this phrase but spoke more separately of their relationships with partners and children, both having decided to have children first, then later married or cohabited. One described her decision to marry:

> I wouldn't, even if I'd reached 25 and didn't have a baby, I wouldn't marry. I'm the type of person who believe you should have a baby before you marry because for me child is important. . . . If I couldn't have any kids, I don't see the point in me getting married, that's how I look at it anyway. (RD)

Although she also described marriage as 'the natural thing to do', she separated it both in time and mind from mothering. This orientation may entail less conflicting values when faced with a choice between partner and child on the discovery of sexual abuse. If it is significantly associated with race, it is one possible explanation for the finding of an earlier study that black children who were sexually abused were more likely than white children to be believed and supported by their mothers. However, it is equally possible that this is attributable to the relationship of the perpetrator since black children were less likely to have been abused by biological fathers than white children (Pierce and Pierce, 1984, cited in Faller, 1988b). It is also possible that orientations to marriage have more to do with the incidence of male unemployment than race per se. Women are less likely either to marry or cohabit with their male partners if their partners are unemployed (Phoenix, 1991) and unemployment is higher amongst Afro-Caribbean than white men. Another study suggested that findings which suggested race differences – in this case that ethnic minority mothers were somewhat more likely to be punitive to their children than white mothers – could be due to poverty and stress, as well as possibly to different attitudes to child-rearing (Gomes-Schwartz *et al.*, 1990). The possibility that such a value orientation is associated with race and reduces conflict should not be taken to reinforce the stereotype of strong, all-coping Afro-Caribbean women.[1]

The relationship of the abuser to the child also affected women's responses. In the context of child-rearing as an ongoing site of marital conflict, women had slightly more leverage with stepfathers than with biological fathers, since against the former they could say 'She's my daughter and I'll say'. In cases with biological fathers, this source of authority was removed, although clarity about the sexual abuse as wrong re-established it for EJ: 'He had constantly told me that I had no business interfering between him and his daughter . . . but over that one particular I thought I had, but over a lot of other things I thought I hadn't.' This may in part account for Faller's (1988a) finding that women still living with the child's biological father were less able to protect the child from abuse than women living with stepfathers/live-in partners, since shared parenthood may reduce their leverage in an unequal relationship.

The way in which men and mothering are combined varies over the life cycle, and the length of time women have already been with an abusive partner and the anticipated length of time that the child will remain in their care are part of the context of their response. Number of years in a relationship has been found significant in women's decisions to leave a relationship abusive to themselves (Strube and Barbour, 1983). The longer the relationship the more the investment may have to be justified by staying, contributing to entrapment. However, a long relationship may also be a deteriorating one, and in the present study this was a counterbalancing influence, resulting in no clear connection between decisions to separate and length of relationship.

Similarly, it is not possible to establish a connection between the age of the child and response. One study has found that younger children were more likely to be believed (Sirles and Franke, 1989) and their mothers were more likely to divorce (Sirles and Lofberg, 1990). However, while young children may have closer relationships with their mothers, they also indicate a longer period ahead of caring for a victimised child (possibly alone) which may influence decisions. Two women also referred to the fact that children left you anyway, whereas husbands were expected to stay for life. Fear of the 'empty nest' syndrome may thus influence response, especially with an older child.

Perceived options for remarriage were an issue for ten women (including one whose relationship had ended shortly after the discovery of abuse although her partner was not himself the abuser), and one that was complicated for most by the effects of the abuse on themselves and/or the child. The value attached to remarriage varied according to stage in the life cycle, the way in which men and mothering were combined and the woman's economic options, but only one expressed no desire for a further relationship. In general, the greater the value attached to remarriage, the more ambivalence resulted from the conflict that might or did arise between the abused child and a new partner.

Economic status

The relationship of women's economic status to their response to a child's sexual abuse has received relatively little attention in research. Two studies have considered it, with conflicting findings. Pellegrin and Wagner (1990) found women were more supportive of their children if they were employed themselves than if they were not, and that children were more likely to be removed from home where their mothers were not in paid employment than if they were. Sirles and Lofberg (1990) did not find women's employment status significant in their decisions to divorce. More attention has been paid to economic factors in research on women's decisions to leave partners violent to themselves. This indicates that women who lack the economic means to establish independent living arrangements are more likely to remain with their partners (Strube, 1988).

It is difficult to establish whether economic dependence was a significant factor in objective terms in the present study, partly because of the size of the sample. In addition, if employment outside the home is taken as an indicator, as it is by Strube and Barbour (1983), this may attribute more 'independence' than is real to women, such as AN, who worked outside the home but whose husband assumed total control over her earnings.[2] Similarly, the small degree of independence women may achieve (as FP and RD in this study did) through homework may be discounted. It seems reasonable to assume, however, that any source of income other than the abusive man lessens dependence to some degree.

Both the women still living with abusive partners at the time of the interviews were wholly dependent on them financially, although one had been working full-time herself at the time of the discovery, but had later given up her job to be at home twenty-four hours a day hoping that this would help to prevent the child being taken into care. All those women (six) who had and maintained a source of independent income, however small, did leave their abusive partners. Three women who were fully economically dependent also separated, although one remarried within six months.

In subjective terms, there were two different ways in which women described money influencing their decisions to leave, distinguished along class lines. The two middle-class women whose husbands abused their children both talked of their economic status in terms of the effects on their dependence/independence. The working-class women however talked more in terms of the effects of money on the state of the marital bargain.

BM had been married for twenty-three years at the time of the interview and had been economically dependent throughout her marriage, bar a short period of part-time work in a factory in the early years. She was middle class in terms of her family background, her own occupation before marriage and her marriage. She had never enjoyed working before her marriage, and marriage and mothering had provided her with an alternative to paid work. She had therefore decided to have a large, well-spaced family in order to stay at home. Cohen (1977) found this pattern common amongst wives of upwardly mobile young executives who, given the alternative of low-status local jobs, often chose pregnancy and the extension of the caring phase rather than face re-entry into the labour market. Similarly, taking on the care of an elderly relative may provide some women with an alternative to paid employment, an option that would not be conceivable for men (Ungerson, 1987).

While BM felt herself lucky in not having to work outside the home and was grateful to her husband for being a good provider, knowing she would be poorer if she were on her own with the children, she missed having any source of income of her own and described clearly the effects of her years of economic dependence on her sense of options:

> I mean I've been dependent on him for so long, and I'd hate to have to
> go to work and support myself. I wouldn't mind having to go, if I had

the sort of job I liked doing and I wouldn't have to make a lot of money out of it, it wouldn't be so bad, but to have to go out to work just to keep body and soul together, I would hate that. . . . 'Cos I've got so dependent on him for everything you see, for everything I am, for what I eat and drink and wear, it all has to come from him, even if I want to buy him a present it has to come out of his money. I don't know, it doesn't bear thinking about. (BM)

EJ had been economically dependent on her husband for ten years while she brought up four children. Again, middle class herself in all senses, she had not felt able to leave the marriage, despite physical, psychological and sexual violence to herself, partly because of her economic status. By the time she discovered her daughter's abuse she had retrained as a teacher and been working for a year and felt that this enabled her to consider leaving:

You see, prior to that I hadn't any real qualifications and really, no means of earning a living as such. . . . I think that it did something to me. Because I was actually not just mixing with housewives and mothers and people who were doing, putting up with the same sort of thing, you know, the usual domestic bit when not all of them wanted to. . . . I think it sort of helped, the fact that I could earn a living, which was not as much as my husband's, but there were men on the staff who could keep a wife and children on the kind of salary that I was getting. (EJ)

These two examples illustrate the effects of paid work and economic independence on self-worth, as well as on material options. Given the significance of paid work in protecting women with children against depression (Brown and Harris, 1978), the connection found between father–daughter incest and depressed mothers is likely to operate by restricting women's options to leave abusive or potentially abusive situations.

Four women in the study, all from working-class backgrounds, had been the breadwinners for their families themselves (three in low-paid, unskilled, part-time jobs and one in full-time clerical work), while their husbands were long-term sick or unemployed. The significance for them of their wage-earning was less concerned with 'independence' – a concept of limited relevance given the low level of their wages and, for one, her husband's control over them – than with its contribution to their sense of betrayal at the discovery that, while they had been out at work, their husbands had been abusing their children. Two expressed the significance of money in their decisions to separate in terms of feeling cheated, their marriages having become a very bad bargain, in which they did everything and got nothing in return, rather than in terms of independence. It was in this context that PE, having supported her partner for many years while he was out of work, and with him in full-time work again at the time she discovered the abuse, decided to 'use him for his money' for a while, giving up work herself to protect the child but getting him to pay the mortgage until he got fed up and left.

Social support

Given the fear of being alone expressed by many women and the traumatic and stigmatised nature of the circumstances, support from others outside the immediate family was also an important influence on the women's decisions to stay or leave. Studies of divorce suggest that supportive links with parents after marriage offer some protection from divorce (Thornes and Collard, 1979). However, where child sexual abuse is involved and divorce becomes a positive rather than negative outcome, it seems that this factor may work in reverse – that is to say, the support that enables women to hold together a marriage in some circumstances may also enable them to leave it when the need arises. Studies of women leaving partners violent to themselves confirm both the importance of social support and the common difficulty women experience in finding the help they need (McGibbon *et al.*, 1989; Hoff, 1990). Female friends and relatives appear to be the most common sources approached (McGibbon *et al.*, 1989).

The two women who had stayed long term with husbands who had abused their children both pointed out the significance of their isolation from alternative sources of support. BM commented that her mother's death before she had married had increased her dependence on her husband from the start, comparing herself with other women who commonly receive help from their mothers after childbirth whereas she had received criticism from both her husband and his mother with whom they initially lived. CL, who described the state of her marriage in the aftermath of the abuse as being 'like a brick wall between us', yet valued her husband being around 'because I've got no one else'. Her relationships with her family of origin had involved a great deal of conflict and they had rejected her totally after the abuse was discovered.

Of those women who separated from abusive partners, either before or in response to the discovery of abuse, all except two had close and supportive relationships either with a relative or with friends outside the family, to whom they confided their plans to separate and from whom they got practical help, although they had not always told of the child's abuse. The two who did not have such sources of support, both in regular but conflict-ridden contact with their own mothers, had both had relationships with other men before separating from their husbands, which had helped to overcome their fear of being alone. Both also wanted to be independent and did not move straight into another cohabiting relationship, but had gained from these relationships a sense of other options.

MG had started a new relationship before she discovered the child's abuse, when her husband was imprisoned for another offence. She described this as helpful in overcoming her ambivalence about separating despite his violence against her:

> But when he actually went to prison I thought good, this is it now, this is the final break so I had no choice but be on my own, I didn't like it at first but then after a while I was sort of, well I'm happy now on my own, 'cos I've got really independent now . . . when I had no choice, when he was in the nick, I thought oh this is really good, and I started going out. And I haven't stopped since! (MG)

Her husband had repeatedly told her, in his attempt to secure control over her, that with three children under five, no one else would have her. Going out with other men while he was in prison proved him wrong. This indicates one limitation to the argument commonly put about the negative impact of imprisonment on 'the family' (Glaser and Spencer, 1990).

Given the social context in which marriage and family are for the majority of women their main career and expected to meet all needs for affection and community, it is not surprising that some women, especially those without a sense of belonging to their families of origin or other sources of support, explore options for a new marital relationship before leaving their marriages. As Gordon (1989) suggests, the more powerless the woman, the more likely that only another lover can provide a way out of an abusive marriage. Social isolation is an important source of powerlessness, and it has often been noted that families in which father–daughter incest has occurred are unusually socially isolated (Finkelhor, 1979; Russell, 1984). This study suggests that it is the quality of the social networks that contribute to powerlessness as well as the quantity of contacts.

THE CONTEXT OF RESPONSE: MALE DOMINANCE AND WOMEN'S PSYCHOLOGY

The situation women face on the discovery of sexual abuse by a family member may raise extreme conflicts between former obligations and relationships. The accounts of the women interviewed suggested that women's psychological development in a male-dominated society is significant in understanding the difficulties some women experience in making a choice in such a situation, to the extent that some are immobilised and unable to take any action.

Carol Gilligan (1982) has argued that women have commonly been judged (and found wanting) against a model of decision making in situations of moral conflict derived from the psychological development of men. She suggests that, while men commonly appeal to rules, a hierarchy of rights and an ethic of justice when faced with conflict, women tend to adopt a more pragmatic and contextualised approach, based on an ethic of care, in which rules may be bent in the interests of preserving relationships over time. Gilligan's argument has been criticised for extrapolating from one particular group of women to present an ahistorical (if not essentialist) notion of woman and for emphasising differences between men and women at the expense of overlap and greater complexity to imply a dichotomous view of the two sexes, fixed in eternal opposition (Eichler, 1988; Scott, 1988). Her argument has also sometimes been read as implying that women have some innate moral superiority to men. It is not intended to use her model in such a way here.

If women do adopt an 'ethic of care' this is hardly surprising given contemporary social organisation. As Graham has argued, 'caring defines both the identity and the activity of women in Western society' (1983, p. 30). It is because of that social organisation – the devaluation of caring represented by the low (or no) pay it attracts and the economic dependency it entails for women – that the 'ethic of care' is not wholly positive but entails tensions and contradictions for women and their dependants. As Sapiro puts it, 'Women are defined as individuals who place themselves second. The irony is that this "altruism" often keeps them from helping not only themselves but others they would wish and feel obligated to help' (1990, p. 51). It is possible also that there would be similarities in men's responses faced with a similar situation of conflict. People commonly make judgements in the family arena on different bases from those in the public sphere, adopting particularistic rather than universalistic criteria. It should also not be assumed that women's thinking about morality follows similar lines in all contexts. If women express the hope that 'in morality lies a way of solving conflicts so that no one will be hurt' (Gilligan, 1982, p. 65), this is likely to be related at least partly to status rather than gender per se. Women in positions of power (as parents, for example) commonly appeal to rules (Hare-Mustin, 1987). In conflicts with men, however, women usually have more to lose. It is in the context of their lack of power in society and dependence on men that they express diffidence, an unwillingness to deal with choice and a tendency to avoid confrontation. It is also this context that makes the conflicts women face when a child is sexually abused by another family member particularly intense.

Women in the present study commonly described themselves as unconfident and their descriptions of their response often demonstrated uncertainty as to the validity of their judgement of the situation and hence to appropriate action, an uncertainty which had frequently been manipulated and exploited by the abusers. The desire not to cause harm (to the abuser, the abused child, other children and other relatives, in varying degrees of priority over time) was a recurring theme in their accounts, impossible though this became in most circumstances. Fear of conflict leaves women unprepared for a situation in which someone has to be hurt and it is their role to pick the victim.

The fear of causing harm does not of course mean that women avoid causing it. On the contrary, reluctance to face conflict may seriously inhibit women from meeting their children's needs where they are being sexually abused by another family member. There is also an apparent contradiction. Alongside the fear of causing harm, there were expressions of homicidal rage and an attempted murder. These are likely however to be linked. The injunction not to harm and fear of conflict that permeates everyday thinking, along with a sense of powerlessness to influence events, may lead to situations so desperate that only violent measures seem feasible or uncontrollable rage is expressed without calculated intention. While care and concern for others may, as Gilligan (1982) argues, have a positive side, this is likely to be the case only where women have enough self-worth to recognise their own needs and agency as well as the conflicting needs of others and to approach choice on that basis.

There were three broadly distinct approaches to choice discernible in these women's accounts. These reflected different approaches to the relationship between the needs of self and others. Some spoke only or primarily in terms of their own survival (although masked behind an image of selflessness). Others expressed anxiety about the 'selfishness' of their motivations, reflecting a desire to be selfless and 'good'. Others (a small minority) spoke openly of balancing their own needs with those of their children and others. These distinctions follow Gilligan's (1982) analysis of women's psychological development. She argues that as women develop a more complex understanding of the relationship between self and other, they are able critically to reinterpret the conflict between selfishness and responsibility that conventional femininity imposes. Hence, their moral judgement moves through a sequence of three perspectives, from concern with survival to concern with goodness to concern with the truth of their own agency and needs. Transition between these perspectives hinges on the development of their own self-worth. The injunction to care that permeates women's moral thinking has to be extended to include care for self in order to achieve responsibility for choice. 'Once obligation extends to include the self as well as others, the disparity between selfishness and responsibility dissolves' (Gilligan, 1982, p. 94).

Each of the three approaches is discussed and illustrated below. They are stages in a process along which women may progress and/or regress and it is not therefore intended to place each woman categorically in relation to her psychological development. Within each approach, a range of different outcomes in relation to an abusing partner and abused child are possible. This conceptualisation offers a more complex and dynamic framework for understanding response than the apparently static typology sometimes adopted of self-, child- or offender-orientated responses (de Francis, 1969). Again it is worth noting that such distinctions may well be present in the moral thinking of men too, and they are not adopted here as essentially female, but because they pointed to differences in the ways in which these women understood and approached the situation and in the significance of the notion of choice to them.

Surviving

It is frequently noted that many women, when the sexual abuse of a child by their partners is disclosed to agencies, are more concerned with the effects of the abuse on their own lives than on their children's. It has also been argued that those women who stay with partners who are sexually abusing their daughters and tell no one are implicitly saying to the child: 'For my own survival, I must leave you to your own devices' (Herman and Hirschman, 1977, p. 746).

The majority of the women in this study talked of their response and decisions primarily in terms of their own survival although this did not necessarily rule out concern for the child's needs and in no case did it mean they were indifferent to the abuse. On the contrary, for women whose very limited self-worth derived largely from their family roles, the losses involved in the discovery of abuse could be particularly devastating, reducing their resources to respond in any mode other than survival. Nor did their concern with their own survival mean that they all stayed with abusive partners as their own survival sometimes dictated that they left as other options arose or as the costs of the marriage became intolerable.

LH's story is perhaps the most extreme example of a woman whose sense of loss at the sexual abuse of her daughter by her husband combined with her low self-worth made her own needs too overwhelming to consider the perspective of others at all. Her response was discussed briefly in Chapter 3 but is introduced again here to illustrate a survival-orientated response. LH perceived the relationship between her husband and her daughter as a love affair, for which both were equally to blame since both had denied it to her and her daughter had herself suggested, at the age of 18, that LH leave the home, which she did three years later. She felt rejected by both of them and, though she dated her 'knowledge' varyingly back to her daughter being between 14 and 16, she was still seeking proof five years after leaving the home.

Her response to her suspicions had been alternately to seek proof and to fight for her own survival, staying out of the house as much as possible and at the same time continuing to perform her role as she saw it:

> I used to just go in and do the shopping, make sure he's got a packet of cigs every day, make sure he doesn't need any shirts nor socks, make sure everything was clean, did all the jobs, but every night I used to work till half past six, and then, I was on six while ten, but I always used to find somewhere to go because I couldn't stand to be in with him, you know. (LH)

She had confronted her daughter with questions such as 'Why are you following your dad? Why don't you come out with me any more?' and 'Why do you have to have sex with your dad? Why don't you go and get a boyfriend, why spoil my life?' She saw herself entirely as a victim, one who had looked after others all her life and been repaid with ingratitude and rejection.

When her daughter became pregnant at 16, despite her rage at this 'proof' of their relationship, which both her husband and her daughter continued to deny, she looked after the baby too, expressing her own needs indirectly in an excess of (not always appropriate) giving:

> I thought well the poor soul's not asked to be born . . . I worked like mad, because she was having a baby, and I bought her a pram. He had everything, when that child was born . . . he wanted for nothing, I can promise, he even had his own toothbrush and he wasn't even born . . . all my wages went on baby things. (LH)

She was aware that this response would be interpreted by others as condoning the relationship but that was certainly not her perception of it and she continued to fight with her husband and daughter while finding some consolation in looking after the baby.

When she finally left the home, she did not see it as a choice but spoke with bitterness of the house she had left behind of which she had been proud, and of her husband helping her out of the house. Leaving represented a defeat to her, and she talked of having stayed so long with no guilt, 'five years I stuck it', as her way of resisting rejection and clinging to a sense of herself as someone who could keep her family together. She seemed to have been enabled to leave largely by starting new relationships with men which had given her back some small sense of self-worth and helped to overcome her fear of being alone.

LH had been the eldest girl in her own family of origin and been the carer of all her seven siblings. Her mother had opposed her marriage, wanting her to continue this role, and, although she had married and left home, she had continued for many years to visit her mother every day to look after her and her younger siblings, and still continued to visit her mother regularly although she felt continually rejected by her mother and able to visit only if she took presents.

The limited self-worth she had gained in her life relied primarily on her marriage, which had seemed to offer a way out of poverty and deprivation. When she met her husband at eighteen, she thought he was

> smashing . . . I mean they had a telly and they had a car, and I mean I'd never had a telly I thought it was posh . . . I'd never even had a carpet, we had board in our bedrooms, I mean I scrubbed boards, we had coats on our beds, us lot. (LH)

Having become pregnant without knowing how, she 'had to get married' but enjoyed it primarily for the social status it gave her: 'I loved being married . . . we had a smashing life, I mean everybody used to envy me, you know, everybody used to say ooh I wish I had a husband like hers.'

She had had seven children herself, of whom three had died, and had poor health, but she prided herself on having been a good mother and on always keeping herself smart looking. Her devastation at her sense that her daughter had both turned against her and robbed her of her marriage, and at the loss of her marriage, a threat to her self-worth compounded by a psychiatrist who suggested that her husband had needed a younger figure as a result of her ageing, left her with no resources to think beyond her own needs, which she continued to express through compulsive looking after others. Although she was aware that her daughter who was still living with her father was not happy, she hated both of them and wished them dead. Despite her active responses, in terms of choice she had been immobilised by her own struggle for survival.

Doing the right thing

Three women talked of their dilemmas more in terms of goodness than survival, expressing concern over what was the right thing to do, lack of confidence in their own judgement of the situation and anxiety about their own needs. In this context the judgements of others became extremely important and could either induce further conflict and guilt or facilitate action if they provided backing for the mothers' own judgements and needs. The first outcome was illustrated by a woman (AN) caught between conflicting messages when her child returned to live with her after eighteen months in care and her disturbed and demanding behaviour brought difficulties in her new relationship. One professional involved was telling her that 'this child needs her mother', that she must reassure the child that she was back with her for good and that, if she lost her relationship, it was not worth much anyway. Another, who she felt knew her better, said that she would not be happy as a lone parent, that the child perhaps needed someone with greater strength than AN who had been psychologically abused, raped and harassed herself by her husband and that for her own sake she should consider letting the child go. These different messages exacerbated the conflict with which she was struggling between selfishness and responsibility, and she expressed her own ambivalence about the child and sense of her needs with great difficulty.

The alternative outcome, in which the judgements of others facilitated action by incidentally legitimating the mother's own needs at the same time as instructing her in relation to the child's, is illustrated by EJ. EJ's account of her attempts to leave her husband when she discovered his abuse of her daughter, a process which took a year from discovery to separation, illustrates her concern with goodness as defined by others, as well as her fear of a violent husband. Her initial response was to threaten to leave her husband, but after he threatened her with murder of the whole family, she retracted, persuading him to go to a psychiatrist instead, hoping that the psychiatrist would 'tell him to get lost . . . because I couldn't do it and make it work on my own'. The psychiatrist's disbelief of her and support for her husband left her 'defeated' and it was not until a year later, when she took her daughter to see the Medical Officer at school, who said 'you must get her away' and also a solicitor who told her she could have him prosecuted that she was able to decide to leave. Both these incidents made her feel that she was right to go and, together with the child's trust in her to sort it out, that she was not alone. Her self-worth was enhanced by this response allowing her to trust her own judgement: 'I felt as though I could do something right for once.'

She talked of being brought up in a strict and respectable middle-class home with a strong emphasis on pleasing others and on doing 'the right thing'. Later in life she had come to realise that what was right in some circumstances was not in others, but at the time she discovered the abuse:

> I had to be doing the right thing, and I think I hadn't left before because I felt I hadn't got sufficient reason to do so. . . . I didn't know what the right thing was to do, the right thing to do was to make my marriage work. That was the right thing to do. And I think that suddenly seeing that it wasn't the right thing to do, to stay, decided me to go. (EJ)

EJ felt guilty about the year it had taken her to leave, insisting that 'you always have a choice' and that she was responsible for her actions. She still however expressed anxiety about the 'selfish' motivations which she felt had allowed her to leave. She had never doubted her daughter's word about the abuse but said 'maybe I wanted something big enough, you know, for a reason to leave'. Despite fifteen years in a marriage to a man who was jealous and possessive, and physically, sexually and psychologically abusive to her, her recognition of her own need to leave was expressed in a self-deprecating fashion through insistence on her selfishness (a clearly negative concept):

> I didn't know what to do. I felt panicky, but to be honest I was selfish in that I thought I've really got something on him now. . . . You know, it was selfish because I felt that all my efforts, in every direction, had gone for nothing. (EJ)

In the context of feminine virtue as self-sacrifice, the protection of the child provided a new moral imperative to leave, whereas the protection of herself from her husband's violence had never done so. Once she had made the decision however, the relief it brought her overcame her anxiety about her own needs since there was no longer a conflict between them and 'doing the right thing':

> I didn't have this sort of torment, am I doing the right thing or should I do that, or if I do so and so will such and such happen or, you know, I had all that going on before, and all of a sudden that stopped you see, which was, which made it easy. (EJ)

Working it out

The transition to full responsibility for choice involves an acknowledgement of the needs of self as equal to those of others and the overcoming of the apparent conflict conventional femininity imposes between selfishness and responsibility. Only two mothers in this study had achieved the necessary self-worth to talk clearly, if somewhat defiantly, about working out what they wanted for themselves, at the same time as taking responsibility for their daughters' protection and rebuilding their relationships with them.

PE's account illustrates an approach to decision making which accorded equal value to her own needs and the child's, and which demonstrates the positive role of an 'ethic of care' in resolving conflicting relationships. She decided not to report her partner to the police when she confirmed his abuse for several reasons. She did not wish to hurt him, feeling he needed help. She wanted both to protect the child from further abuse and to rebuild her own relationship with her, and felt that involving the police against the child's expressed wishes would further damage her trust. She also felt she still loved her partner and wanted to work out what she wanted for herself. She first separated her partner and child and rebuilt her relationships with both – arranging for the child to stay with friends and visiting her every day – then later when she felt her own relationship with her partner had improved, brought the child home, trusting her partner's promises of reform.

As he then continued to attempt to sexually abuse the child and, thwarted by her protection, became physically violent to R, the conflict between the two relationships became irreconcilable, and she started to hate him. 'When he started to become violent towards her, that was it. He wrote his own sentence out as far as I was concerned.' And she decided to 'get rid of him'. She had eventually done so, and had achieved what she wanted, a close and confiding relationship with her daughter again and no regrets over separating from her partner. She did not talk with guilt of having stayed this six months, although she did express anxiety – 'I know this might sound terrible' – at having decided to use her partner for his money for a while and try to get him to leave rather than kick him out immediately and risk losing the house because she would not be able to pay the mortgage payments. She felt however that she had made her own choices, attending to both her own needs and the child's throughout:

> I thought I loved him, which I didn't. I was scared of losing my home, my daughter and that was it. And I didn't quite know how to keep it all together, and that was the only way I knew how. And that's what I done. And it did work out, I mean what I done did work out right. (PE)

Working through this process meant that it took her six months from confirming the abuse to separating from the abuser. She was clear that had she done 'the right thing' as defined by others, that is, called the police immediately, she would not have stood a chance of regaining the child's trust, which had been badly damaged by the abuse, nor would she have been able to work out for herself what she wanted with her partner.

This approach is reminiscent of a woman quoted by Gilligan who, seeing the world as comprised not of separate individuals with competing rights but as an interconnected network of relationships in which 'the fact that someone is hurt affects everyone who is involved', describes a moral decision as one which involves working through everything involved in the situation and taking responsibility for choice:

> It is taking the time and energy to consider everything. To decide carelessly or quickly or on the basis of one or two factors when you know that there are other things that are important and that will be

affected, that's immoral. The moral way to make decisions is by considering as much as you possibly can, as much as you know.

(Gilligan, 1982, p. 147)

The implications of the range of approaches presented here are twofold. First, delays in taking action when the abuse of a child is discovered may be the product of quite different processes. The woman may have been immobilised by her own struggle for survival and unable to consider action to protect her child. Alternatively she may have been confused over what the right thing to do was in the context of the conflicting needs of others and her own conflicting obligations, and have been further inhibited by lack of confidence in her own judgement and/or ambivalence about her own needs. Or, finally, she may have been working through the conflicts between her own needs and those of others, attempting to find a solution which reconciles the relationships involved. It is important to recognise the different processes since instructions from professionals in relation to the child's needs will have a different impact depending on the meaning choice has for the mother. Women preoccupied with surviving may resist intervention as a further threat to their own identity as mothers. Those confused about what the right thing to do is are likely to be more receptive to intervention, which however may reinforce anxiety and confusion if it focuses only on their responsibilities. Alternatively it may facilitate choice if the woman's own needs are recognised (deliberately or accidentally). Women who have been working out the conflicting relationships may resist intervention if professionals fail to recognise the integrity of their own process of response.

Second, choice has little meaning to women in these circumstances unless they have some sense of their own self-worth, the legitimacy of their own needs and of their agency and power to influence events. Those who were immobilised, that is, those who expressed no sense of having made a choice, were those preoccupied with their own survival in the face of loss. Immobility in relation to choice, like failure to confirm in relation to discovery, is linked to the inability to resolve the grieving process (see Chapter 3). Becoming stuck in unresolved grief inhibited women both from resolving the discovery process and from making choices. Hence, their own needs for self-worth and empowerment should as far as possible be met before long-term choices are expected. While this is a small sample and the distinctions not clear-cut, it suggests that those women with a clear sense of their own needs as legitimate as well as the child's were more likely to choose to separate from an abusive partner than those without.

THE PROCESS OF RESPONSE

The process of response women engaged in has four central features. First, they tended to consider a far wider network of relationships than the abuser and the child, and to perceive the problem as one of conflicting relationships and responsibilities extending over time rather than one of separate individuals in a hierarchy of competing rights. Second, ongoing processes of negotiation and mediation meant that their response changed as one or more elements of the situation changed, the perceived risk to the child, their own relationships with the abuser or others, or the success or failure of earlier attempts to resolve the situation. Third, the process of attempting to reconcile potentially and actually conflicting relationships necessarily involved a degree of risk taking. Fourth, most attempted to resolve conflict via communication-based strategies, at least initially.

To illustrate the process, one relatively straightforward case in which the woman had no significant relationship herself with the abusers, who were not members of the same household as the child, is outlined below. JT's 5-year-old daughter K was abused in two separate incidents, both times while in the care of her father from whom JT was separated. The father, S, was now living with his sister and her children and took K to their house when he had access visits with her. The first incident occurred there, and the abuser was K's 13-year-old cousin, a boy whom JT described as 'backward' with a mental age of 6, and who, she knew, had been sexually abused himself. She also knew that the boy had a social worker, and she first tried to contact the social worker, who, she felt, should be able to deal with the boy. Since she was unable to do so, she then told his mother, who agreed to deal with it, and felt that the situation had been 'sorted out'. She had been shocked and distressed by the discovery but her knowledge of the boy's problems affected her response, 'because I knew that he'd got a problem . . . I seemed to sort of cope with it'. She reassured K that it would not happen again.

However, shortly after, K was abused again in similar circumstances (while in the care of her father) by the boy's older brother. This time JT was more angry and distressed and gave three reasons in explaining why this incident was worse. First, the abuser's characteristics were different, and hence his responsibility for his own actions different: 'He was 15 so I mean he knew what he was doing and there was nothing wrong with him, you know.' Second, her own relationship with her daughter felt threatened – she had told K that it would not happen again and it had. She had not been able to prevent it and felt the child's trust in her would be damaged. Third, she was furious with her ex-husband for not taking the problem more seriously, for leaving the child unattended with her cousins again and for not sharing her sense of responsibility for preventing the recurrence of abuse.

This time her ex-husband said he would sort it out with the family and JT talked to her health visitor about what had happened, wanting to have K seen by a doctor to check for any physical damage. On the health visitor's advice she also reported the incident to the police, feeling it was right to do so because of his age and the possibility of him doing it to someone else, although she also told the police that 'because he was family' she did not particularly want him to be charged. Via this process she also had contact with a social worker and, with his backing, reassured K that she would never see the abusers again and agreed with her ex-husband that he would prevent this happening. She also spoke again to the abuser's mother who this time did not believe her, thinking she was 'having a go' at the whole family now.

Two months later, her ex-husband took K on an access visit again and although he did not take her to the house where she had been abused, she did see both cousins while out with him. Again, JT was furious with her ex-husband, for his failure to take responsibility for K and for the threat to her own relationship with K, as well as the risk to K herself:

> 'Cos I thought what can I say, what can I say to her, there wasn't anything else to say then, there was nothing left, I couldn't turn round and say you can trust me K, because you know, she trusted me and he still took her . . . luckily enough nothing did happen. (JT)

She was also angry with the social workers involved who had spoken only to her about K and not to her ex-husband, feeling that they should share the responsibility for making him take her protection seriously. Up until this point she had not considered refusing her ex-husband access to K, feeling that he loved her in his way, although he was much less protective than herself, and that K's relationship with her father should be maintained for her to make her own decisions about when she grew up. However she now consulted a solicitor in order to draw up conditions of access and threatened him that if he ever allowed K to see her cousins again, his access would be stopped.

While JT was clear about the need to protect the child from further contact with her abusers, she also worried about the network of family relationships extending into the future. If the child is to go on seeing her father, is she never to see his relatives, her cousins, ever again, and what implications will this have for her relationship with her father?

> What happens, what happens in time, does she see them, does she sort of see them? You know, I mean there are occasions when perhaps there might be something, and he wants to take her to you know, there might be a wedding in the family or something, mightn't there in time? You

know, what does she do, does she never see them again? . . . I mean that's where I wish that they, they hadn't been family because you know, they're always going to be there aren't they, in the background, unless she never sees him again, and what'll happen to her then you know? (JT)

While her concern extends to the maintenance of a network of family relationships over time, her approach is essentially pragmatic, recognising that she can make judgements only on the basis of a particular context, and that the negotiation of conflicting relationships is an ongoing process:

> although I'm thinking of these things, what's going to happen in the future, I sort of think to myself well you're going to have to sort that out when it comes to it, you know. So I'm not sort of desperate or anything, you know, I just, I mean I wonder about it, but I think well you'll have to cope with that when it comes to it, you know, you'll have to sort that out. (JT)

One further incident illustrates the extended network of relationships involved and the way in which within this child-rearing is a risk-taking process. During the investigation process, some confusion had arisen over the identity of K's abuser and JT had raised the possibility of it being her new cohabitee. Although this suspicion was completely cleared up, a social worker had then warned JT not to leave K vulnerable to such a situation arising in the future. She was horrified at the suggestion that she must now be suspicious all the time in her own home and never leave her partner and the child alone together. At first she did feel she could not trust him and tried not to leave them together but after a while started to do so occasionally when she went out to the shops:

> Now I've just sort of . . . put it out of our mind you know, and sort of tried to carry on as a normal family. Because I think you've got to, I mean all right if anything is going to happen, you know, I hope to god it wouldn't ever you know, I hope to god it wouldn't ever . . . that she'd come out with it, you know . . . but I've got to sort of, you know, I've got to trust him and sort of think, you know, that he wouldn't . . . I just don't know if I'm doing the right thing, you know, but I've got no suspicions . . . and B [the cohab] and I do sort of talk honestly and openly and everything. . . . But you know, I just sort of, you have to go each day by day really, you know, I think you've just got to carry on, haven't you, you've got to carry on sort of as a normal life really, and just try and forget about it. (JT)

There is no basis to suggest that this woman was putting her partner above her child by relaxing her vigilance. She was quite clear that she would be devastated if anything at all further happened to the child, and had insisted on checking out fully the suspicions that had fallen on her cohabitee, despite feeling that her 'world was falling apart'. What she was doing afterwards, however, was taking a chance in the interests of maintaining a network of relationships over time, relying on communication to resolve potential conflicts and expecting some shared responsibility for the child's protection with her new partner. Her response throughout involved negotiating her own relationship with the child, the child's relationship with her father, the child's relationship with other relatives, and her own and her daughter's relationships with her new cohabitee, as well as consideration of the relationship between the abusers and her daughter.

The conflict the discovery of abuse by a partner raises between the mother's relationships with the abuser and with the child is far more acute than that in the case described above. Nevertheless, there is similarly a wider network of relationships involved extending over time, including the abuser's relationship with other children, the children's relationships with the mother's new partner if she remarries, the mother's relationships with other children as well as the mother's and her partner's family of origin and other sources of support or conflict. And similarly the process of response, attempting to negotiate potentially and actually conflicting relationships, is an ongoing one. Categorising response by outcome assuming a straightforward choice between child and abuser does not adequately represent the complexity, variability and ongoing nature of mothers' responses. Attributing the recurrence of abuse after the mother's discovery to collusion also assumes that women have information available to them at the beginning of a process, that the abuser will abuse again, that only becomes available at the end.

The rest of this section discusses the process of response for the nine women who discovered abuse by resident partners, only during the period from discovery to separating (or not) from the abusive partner, that is, as they considered the alternatives of attempting to prevent further abuse within the family or separating. During this period particularly, there was an important additional influence on the process – fear: fear of violent repercussions against themselves and/or their children if they confronted their partners and fear of being alone if they left them. Of these nine cases, in five the child was abused again after the mother's discovery. In none of these cases however did the women condone the abuse and three of them had gone to great lengths in their attempts to prevent recurrence, including separating the child and abuser for periods and accompanying the child full-time where possible. Furthermore, in four of these five cases, the women had by the time of the interviews resolved the situation, separating from their partners and maintaining their relationships with their daughters.

In the fifth case, the woman had lost both relationships, finally leaving her husband and daughter still living together.

The inability of some women to prevent recurrence of sexual abuse by family members is better understood as the product of risk taking than as collusion with the abuse itself. PE, who had decided not to inform the police on her initial discovery and been criticised by her sister for not doing so, expressed this:

> She'd have to admit herself what I done sort of worked out right, she said but it could have worked out wrong, I said well that was the chance I took, it was something I had to sort out myself, and I took that chance and it worked out fine.[3] (PE)

Three of these nine women were unable to develop ways of preventing further abuse at all. For those who were not so immobilised, their responses were influenced by their assessment of the risk that the abuse would recur and of the worth of the marriage to them, and their interaction with others outside as well as within the family. Interaction with those outside the household is discussed further in the next chapter. Factors affecting the assessment of the risk of recurrence and the worth of the relationship are discussed here, followed by the issue of responsibility which affects both. As Sgroi (1982) has noted, the ability to be an effective ally for a child depends on allocating responsibility clearly to the abuser.

Women's assessment of the risk of recurrence was influenced by a number of factors: primarily the abuser's response to confrontation, the mother's way of explaining the abuse, her perception of the father–daughter relationship, her sense of her own capacity to protect the child and her knowledge of the extent of abuse. Abusive men who confessed when confronted professed remorse and promised reform. Many mental health professionals working with sexually abusive men (with far less investment in their relationships with them) have been fooled by similar strategies (McGovern and Peters, 1988). Those who denied the abuse nevertheless attempted to win their wives round with promises of better behaviour generally, presents and so forth. Women were reluctant to lose all trust in men they still cared about as well as depended on, although three who hoped for reform did not rely on trust alone to prevent recurrence.

The two who did rely on trust alone both blamed themselves for the abuse. Self-blame suggested that if the woman herself 'did better' in some way, the abuse would not recur. An explanation of abuse as illness on the other hand implied the possibility of a cure, and two women had sought psychiatric help for their partners on that basis. Hopes of reform lasted longer for two who thought their partners had relationships of special favouritism with the children than for one who felt her husband had always been hostile to the child.

Two initially believed (as have many child abuse experts in the past) that 'breaking the secrecy' and rebuilding communication between all parties would prevent the recurrence of abuse. As PE put it, 'I thought once it was out, he'd lay off'. As evidence of their partners' persistence recurred, despite their efforts to restrict access and build closer relationships themselves with their children, their assessment of the situation changed and they sought ways to separate.

Women's assessment of the worth of the marriage to them was influenced by the social, economic and psychological factors discussed earlier in this chapter, and involved reference to love and hate, violence, conflict and fear, and their partner's contribution to the marital bargain. For no woman was her child's abuse the sole reason for separating. The five who made decisions to separate permanently from their partners in response to the discovery of sexual abuse had all considered separating before, either on account of violence against themselves or in one case because of an earlier incident of child sexual abuse, and four had actually done so and returned in the past. This is a common pattern in women's response to domestic violence and other marital problems, recurring hopes and promises of reform, together with self-blame and the desire to make marriages work, bringing women back until the relationship deteriorates further (Dobash and Dobash, 1979; Burgoyne *et al.*, 1987). For all these, the abuse of the child was one of, if not the, 'last straw(s)' in a deteriorating marriage, and separation a relief. Violence to the child gave them a reason to leave in a way that violence to themselves had not, and only one expressed any regret at separating.

The single factor most predictive of decisions to separate was a previous separation. This is consistent with the findings of research on women's decisions to leave relationships violent to themselves, which suggests that those who stay tend to have suffered less severe abuse and to have separated from the abusers less often in the past (Strube, 1988). The 'last straw' factor may also explain Sirles and Lofberg's (1990) finding that previous violence against the mother was significantly related to decisions to divorce.

None of the three women who were immobilised nor the one who considered no further decision was necessary once she had stopped the abuse recurring had ever considered separating from their partners before. These four women's fears were expressed primarily in terms of fear of being alone. 'Company', whatever its quality, and, for two of them, the social acceptability attached to being married appeared to be the overriding benefits of their relationships, illustrating their extremely low expectations and self-worth. Being unmarried for them meant being alone, reflecting the social context in which marriage and family are expected to meet all needs for community and the lack of social value accorded other sources of companionship such as female friendship.

A key factor enabling women to leave abusive partners was a clear sense of the abuser's responsibility for the abuse. While mothers have often been observed to blame children for abuse, self-blame is also a problem. Two of the women who were immobilised still blamed themselves at the time of the interview, as did both women who were still living with the abusive partner. Overcoming self-blame had played an important part in enabling effective action for others.

The question of responsibility was related to the explanations women adopted for the abuse, and confounded by confusions that also permeate public debate: are abusers sick and in need of treatment or criminals deserving of punishment? and are they victims of their childhoods or adults abusing their power? These questions are interrelated and both influence the degree of responsibility accorded abusers for their actions. Illness is generally regarded as outside the individual's control and therefore not deserving of blame, although taking the necessary action to ensure re-covery is seen as the individual's responsibility (Cornwell, 1984). Hence abusers who promised to seek help were accorded diminished responsi-bility until they proved they had no serious intention of doing so. Illness also implies the possibility of cure and hence affected women's judgement of future options. Similarly the abuser's own childhood experiences of abuse or violence also diminished responsibility either via a disease model or by shifting the responsibility back a generation. One woman (not in this nine) referred to abuse by a boy who had been sexually abused himself as his own experience 'coming out', rather like a rash. Another blamed her husband's mother for his difficult childhood.

While such explanations may diminish responsibility and those women who focused on conscious action ('he knew what he was doing') and the moral responsibility ('old enough to know right from wrong') attached to adult status were clearer about the individual abuser's responsibility, they do imply individual as opposed to family explanations. The adoption of familial explanations based on patriarchal ideas about marriage and the family were major sources of guilt and confusion over responsibility, which clearly inhibited action. There were three main variations on these. First, the 'he wasn't getting enough' explanation, when accompanied by assumptions of men's rights to sexual access in marriage, induced self-blame where the abuser was the woman's partner. Second, the idea that women are the rightful monitors of all family relationships through their 'natural' aptitude for caring left one woman unable to allocate responsi-bility for any family problem clearly to her husband. Third, another woman blamed herself and had been blamed by others for going out to work and leaving her husband to look after her children, an explanation clearly relying on ideas of a patriarchal sexual division of labour as 'natural'. The absence of her partner at work could never seriously be suggested as an explanation for a mother abusing her child.

Only one woman blamed her daughter explicitly, partly because the child, a teenager of about 15 when LH's suspicions first arose, had appeared to her not only not to resist but to defend the relationship with her father by denying it when questioned. Children's delay in telling about abuse has been found to increase the likelihood of negative responses from their mothers (Gomes-Schwartz *et al.*, 1990). Others also commonly attribute blame to children who have not resisted abuse (Broussard and Wagner, 1988). In two other cases, women expressed some ambivalence in the observation that the abuse would not have happened if the child had not been there. Women commonly blame themselves for their own experiences of sexual violence on the basis of 'being there', demonstrating the power of the discourse which holds women responsible for male violence (Kelly, 1988a). The significance of this dominant discourse is further indicated by evidence that mothers tend to be more protective and less punitive when the victimised child is a son than a daughter (Gomes-Schwartz *et al.*, 1990). One recent study found that in two cases where children of both sexes in the same family had been abused, the mothers regarded the girls but not the boys as culpable (Dempster, personal communication, 1990). There are also cases of sibling incest in which abused daughters are blamed by their mothers for the behaviour of their brothers (La Fontaine, 1990). Unless this discourse is challenged and alternative ways of understanding abuse offered, the options women face where abuse by partners is concerned are likely to be blaming themselves or their children.

While self-blame for the abuse itself was immobilising, those women who were most able to take action emphasised their own responsibility for their response. To some extent this is a form of self-blame, which comes down ultimately to 'being her mother', but one which may have a more positive and enabling function once responsibility for the abuse itself is clearly located with the abuser. Self-blame for 'being her mother' on one level reflects the avoidance of male responsibility for sexual violence and for child protection. On another, examining their own behaviour (for example, wishing they had stood up to their husbands more strongly, been less trusting of them or been more aware of the children) also provided a way of considering changes they could make to lessen the risk of the situation recurring. This process of examining their own behaviour however carried the risk of being highly destructive unless culpability for the abuse itself had first been resolved. The issue of self-blame is complex. The total absence of recognition of their own behaviour as an issue left women only with the status of victims and no sense of being able to effect change in their own lives and their children's. However, the timing of such self-examination is crucial. It can only be enabling after responsibility for the abuse itself is clearly located with the abuser and the guilt associated with loss for mothers resolved.

Allocating responsibility for the abuse clearly to the abuser, while it helped to enable separation, did not necessarily reflect an understanding of the nature of abuse. As discussed in Chapter 4, for some women 'abuse' was defined as wrong more in response to sex than in recognition of the abuse of power involved. Two women in this study expressed their aversion to further contact with their partners primarily as a desire to distance themselves from sexual deviance. In this context, separation for one had more to do with the desire to find a better, 'normal' man than to do with the child's need for protection, expressed: 'I mean I won't go with a man that's interfered with my own daughter, I'm not that type of person' (NF). In this context, separation is not necessarily a positive outcome for the child, and her child had been taken into care despite NF having no further contact with the abuser.

SUMMARY AND CONCLUSIONS

Overall, the choice women often face between a child and an abusing partner or other relative is a complex and conflictual matter with long-term implications. Their response is best understood as involving an ongoing process of negotiation and mediation within a network of family relationships. In this process, women take risks in an attempt to reconcile conflicts. The greater the value accorded the marriage (or relationship with an abusive partner) and the fewer the alternative options perceived, the greater the risks that may be taken with the child's safety, but it may well not be possible for women to eliminate all risk of abuse recurring.

Again, there are similarities with the task faced by social workers, who must also negotiate conflicting relationships, with each parent, with children and with substitute carers, in an attempt to preserve a network of relationships over time. The trend in policy has been towards 'legalism', an increasing reliance on rule-bound relationships between workers and clients (Parton and Martin, 1989). Despite strong emphasis on adherence to procedures in the current climate of anxiety however, social workers do not always follow them (Corby, 1987). Several social workers in my study talked of the difficulty of knowing what 'the right thing to do' was in individual cases, one adding that legalistic and procedural responses, with their focus on rules and justice, were inadequate where long-term relationship issues are at stake (Hooper, 1990). For social workers as for mothers the attempt to negotiate conflicting relationships entails the taking of some risks with children's safety.

The analysis in this chapter suggests a number of ways in which women's responses may be influenced. They are more likely to decide to separate from an abusive partner if they perceive the risk of recurrence of abuse to be high. This in turn is more likely if they do not blame themselves for it, but hold the abuser clearly responsible, if they regard it as an intentional act rather than a disease, and as part of a long-term pattern rather than a single, out of character, incident. Where professionals are working with the man who abused the child, passing on to women information about his particular history of offending and the ways in which he groomed the child to ensure continued access can help to clarify these issues. The analogy with addiction may also be useful, offering a way of understanding sexual abuse as an individual rather than familial problem, which retains a sense of the abuser's personal responsibility (since addictions *can* be broken, or at least controlled), alongside the strong likelihood of recurrence. Women are also more likely to separate if they perceive their own relationship with the abuser as unsatisfactory, which in turn depends on self-worth, social and economic resources and the options perceived for (and/or value accorded) remarriage. No woman in this study made the decision to separate on the basis of the child's abuse alone. Hence the empowerment of mothers should not be seen as an alternative to working towards parental responsibility. Rather it is a vital part of such an aim.

It is equally important however that women's past actions are understood in the context of the meaning of the situation to them and their assessment of options at the time. Women's behaviour is often judged only by its outcome and/or against unrealistic expectations. All but one of the women in this study had talked to others outside the family about the abuse prior to their involvement in the research. These interactions as well as those within the family influenced their responses, too often resulting in a sense of invalidation and defeat which inhibited rather than facilitated their ability to protect children. It is this interaction with others outside the family, both in social networks and public agencies, that the next two chapters address.

6 Help-seeking decisions and experience of informal help

Going public where the sexual abuse of a child is suspected or discovered combines many of the difficulties associated with help seeking for other family problems, together with the further complications added by secrecy and conflict within the family and stigma outside it. It is not only fears of prosecution of their partners or of losing their children into care if state agencies become involved (although these may be important factors) that prevent women seeking help. The reluctance of battered women to seek help for themselves reflects cultural ideals of family privacy and results from the sense of shame and guilt consequently involved in admitting to marital problems, pressure from the abusive husband to preserve privacy and expectations of the response of others (Dobash and Dobash, 1979). Battered women often do seek help or leave violent relationships 'for the sake of the children', and for women in the present study the abuse of the child sometimes gave a sense of entitlement to help that they had not felt in relation to their own experiences of violence.

However, for others the abuse of the child also added a further sense of shame and failure on top of the recognition it involved of serious marital problems. Backett's study of middle-class couples found that parents usually went to great lengths to resolve any problems with children within the nuclear group before outside help was sought, and that about a third indicated that to resort to outside advice was 'somehow an admission of failure to cope with something that they should have been able to manage themselves' (1982, p. 102). The difficulty of asking for help is exacerbated both by feelings of personal inadequacy and by a sense of sole responsibility for dependents. Thus, women caring for elderly relatives may feel that asking for help threatens their role as primary carer (Lewis and Meredith, 1988). Similarly, mothers who above all expect themselves to cope (Graham, 1982), experience conflicting feelings about needing help.

This chapter describes first the many factors which the women interviewed felt inhibited their ability to seek help. It is important to consider these in understanding mothers' responses since reporting to agencies is often seen as an indicator of protective behaviour. One study of the attitudes of protective service workers in the USA found that 22 per cent favoured the arrest of the mother in a vignette involving a mother who had delayed reporting her husband's abuse of her daughter (Wilk and McCarthy, 1986). However, as in the case of marital difficulties, women's responses commonly involved a 'help-seeking career' (Brannen and Collard, 1982), and contact with those agencies with statutory duties for child protection was rarely the first attempt to seek help. Most of the women who sought help themselves approached members of their social networks, extended family and friends first. This chapter outlines the aims with which women did seek help, when and from whom, and their experience of informal sources. Voluntary organisations without statutory responsibilities for child protection are included in this chapter. The NSPCC, which does have statutory duties, is included in the next chapter, since its social control function makes it more akin to statutory agencies in relation to the experience of mothers.

FACTORS INHIBITING HELP SEEKING

The factors inhibiting help seeking for the women in this study derived from their own stage in the processes of discovery and decision making, pressures from the reactions of family members, including but not only the child and abuser, their sense of obligation to family members and feelings about the abuse, their expectations and experience of others' reactions outside the family (informal and formal), attitudes to help in general and lack of information about available sources of help.

Clearly, not knowing either that abuse has occurred at all or that it is recurring inhibits seeking help, although two women had sought help for their children's behaviour problems over periods of two and more years without any suspicions arising, either for them or the professionals involved, that sexual abuse might be the cause. Once suspicions of sexual abuse had arisen, women were inhibited from seeking help by their own horror, self-doubt and self-blame at their thoughts. As PE said:

> I thought to myself I must be sick to be thinking anything like it, and I sort of kept it to myself for a little while, until eventually I went and told my, I said to my friend about it. (PE)

In these circumstances women were afraid that others might disbelieve them and/or that if they reported to the police/SSD no action would be taken if there was no proof to substantiate their suspicions. These fears were well justified. Most of the women had experienced disbelief at some point either within their social networks or from professionals even when they did have evidence. Three of the women had contacted agencies about suspicions. In one case an investigation including medical examination found insufficient evidence and despite a case conference no further action was taken. In the other two cases the women were told that nothing could be done without proof.

Visible evidence or a complaint from the child seemed to offer the mother some protection from the anticipated disbelief of others. In the absence of such validation for her own suspicions and concerns, and a reality shared at least with the child, the fear of others' reactions could be overwhelming. Confusion over the definition of abuse further exacerbated the fears attached to lack of proof for KV:

> I didn't feel I had grounds enough to go to the SS, I didn't know what they considered abuse to be. I mean there's abuse which is obviously where a husband, or father, has intercourse with his daughter, I didn't realise there was other degrees of sexual abuse that they would be interested in. (KV)

Ambivalence about confirming suspicions may also inhibit help seeking. Women may both seek the proof to resolve uncertainty and still hope that it will not be forthcoming. A further reason that three women did not seek help was feeling that they had resolved the problem themselves and prevented the abuse recurring and therefore did not need outside help. For one, in addition to this, her expectations of what involving agencies would entail meant that seeking help conflicted with other aims, namely finding out more of what had happened herself, rebuilding the child's trust and taking the time to work through her own feelings and decide what she wanted in relation to her partner. For two women, their understanding of the problem – that their partners were sick and needed help – contributed to their not reporting to the police. Both consulted GPs and arranged for their partners to see psychiatrists.

The factors above derived from the women's own stage of discovery and response. Pressure from others was also important however. Most of those women who confronted their partners with their suspicions or knowledge came under pressure from the men not to tell anyone outside the household, including threats of violence to themselves and the children and various more subtle strategies of manipulation. Fear of violent repercussions meant that two women, when they did seek help, did so secretly. One managed to leave with four children without her husband suspecting anything, but was inhibited from pressing charges for fear that he would spend his time in prison planning revenge. The other confronted her husband after the police and SSD were involved. She informed him of their investigation, but he was unimpressed, replying 'Well, when are you coming home then? I want my dinner.' His judgement of the likely effects of her attempts to seek help proved correct – he denied the allegations and no further action was taken against him.

Two of the children had also specifically asked their mothers not to involve the police when they told them of the abuse, and, having promised them they would not do so, both women were reluctant to betray the children's trust, knowing that it had already been badly damaged by the abuse. Fear of harm to the child, even where no promise was involved, inhibited others from and during help seeking. Some of the children also expressed a desire in the aftermath for no one to know about the abuse, and concern for their privacy inhibited mothers from seeking support for themselves within social networks. One child, on the other hand, told everyone, which left her mother with little privacy.

Pressures came from the involvement of other family members as well, either to protect the abuser by not reporting or to 'clear' him by going through a court case. However, it was not only actual pressures from other family members that influenced women. Their own sense of obligation to family members also inhibited some from reporting to the police and contributed to the sense of unspeakableness surrounding the abuse. Particularistic rather than universalistic role expectations often inhibit the reporting of crimes by family members and even their definition as crimes (Burgess *et al.*, 1977). However, the dilemma this creates is likely to be intensified for mothers in these circumstances by the effects that women's identification with family, rooted in the sexual division of labour and the widely held belief that men and women naturally have different roles, have on women's citizenship. Pateman (1985) has argued that the formal equality of citizenship is contradicted by the current structures of women's subordination whose logic suggests rather that women's political obligation constitutes a duty of obedience acknowledged in the public sphere through the actions of fathers or husbands. In this context, it is not surprising that women may have great difficulty in reporting crimes committed by their husbands/partners to the police. The sense of obligation women had to their partners and their children, and to other family members who might be harmed by going public, contributed to the complexity of feelings surrounding such a decision. For one woman, this resulted in a pattern of help seeking similar to that exhibited sometimes by sexually abused children who attempt to have the abuse discovered but at the same time to disguise their hints.

PE felt unable to report the abuse herself but asked her sister to phone the SSD for her. When they came to visit her, she felt unable to tell them the whole story (involving seven years of abuse, including buggery and rape) but told them her partner was violent and had sexual tendencies towards her daughter:

> I wanted them to find out, I couldn't tell them but I wanted them to tell me, you know well look this has gone on. I couldn't, I felt like I was betraying him and betraying her, and I couldn't open my mouth, I couldn't, it was just stuck there and I couldn't say a word. And I wanted them to say to me, well look, this has gone on in here, and we know it's gone on, but obviously they didn't. (PE)

A case conference was held and she had some continuing contact with the SSD, including taking the child to them when she had been hit by her stepfather and had bruises on her face, but still could not bring herself to tell them about the sexual abuse, wanting them to demand an examination or somehow to take the responsibility for breaking through her own sense that the abuse was unspeakable. She finally called the police herself, after her partner had decided to leave anyway, and had been violent to the child again, but still found it difficult to tell them the full story: 'I just couldn't get it out of my mouth, it was like a bloody lump that was stuck there, I wanted to and it was stuck.' She had however previously been able to tell doctors in hospital who had asked her the reason for a suicide attempt, perhaps finding it easier to speak when out of the home and away from the presence of family members. She also attempted to tell the police by showing a doctor's letter describing what she had told them. When pushed, she did in the end tell the police herself.

The testing tactics and ambivalence that may operate on both sides of the help-seeking relationship reflect the contradictory forces surrounding family violence – the privacy accorded and unity expected of family life on the one hand and the need for public action to prevent violence on the other – within which both professionals and mothers operate.

Obligation to the children also affected decisions about reporting since their future financial security would be affected if their father went to prison. This did not necessarily mean staying with the abusive partner. Although it was a consideration in that decision for one mother (whose own financial security was as influential an inhibiting factor), another divorced but decided not to involve the police partly because she would get no maintenance payments for the children if her ex-husband was unable to earn.

Women's own feelings on finding out about their children's abuse, of shock, confusion, shame, self-blame and isolation, also contributed to not seeking help and to a sense of unspeakableness. Shame, derived from ideals of family privacy (fear of 'hanging the dirty washing out'), from the woman's own relationship with the abuser and associated sense of contamination and from the effects on the child, also continued to influence experience of intervention. RD, whose daughter had had a baby as a result of the abuse, felt ashamed and embarrassed when taking her to the hospital for a post-natal check up: 'I felt if the whole hospital could just open and just push me in it. . . . I felt if they would just open a little bit of ground and pull me through it.' Another woman, whose child was seeing a therapist known to specialise in sexual abuse, was embarrassed that the other mothers waiting at the day hospital had guessed from this that her child had been sexually abused and had pretended to them that there was another reason.

Guilt and self-blame also inhibited some women from seeking help. BM who felt the abuse of her daughter was a responsibility shared between her and her husband did not seriously consider reporting him to the police. To recognise behaviour as criminal involves a concept of personal responsibility which she did not have, although when her husband abused a child outside the family and she consequently attributed responsibility more clearly to him, she was also clearer about considering reporting to the police.

The losses the discovery of sexual abuse involved (especially loss of trust) and the sense often expressed that no one could understand who had not been through this contributed further to ambivalence about help. Several women also said that they had tried to block it out and forget about it in the aftermath and that it was too painful to talk about. Several women had sought and obtained practical help and some emotional support from friends and family without telling them the details of what had happened. As illustrated above with PE's account, it was less possible to achieve any helpful response from agencies in this way.

Expectations of the reactions of others, both in their social networks and agencies, also inhibited mothers from seeking help. They feared disbelief and blame from friends and family. Some also feared that relatives (especially their own mothers) would be shocked and distressed, and sought to protect them by not telling them. Or that others (especially brothers) would be so angry that they would cause further trouble by attacking the abuser personally. They also feared loss of control and privacy if others became involved and did not treat the information as confidential or started telling them what to do and taking over.

Some similar fears inhibited contact with agencies, especially regarding blame, the loss of privacy and control. Class and ethnic background influenced the extra fears and expectations with which women approached or attempted to avoid professionals. Fears of losing the child into care were expressed only by working-class women in this sample, reflecting the reality that children in care come almost exclusively from working-class families (Frost and Stein, 1989). The middle-class women had not thought of this risk at the time of seeking help, although it is likely that events in Cleveland in 1987 have brought more awareness of this possibility to middle-class parents. The middle-class women were less likely to have had any previous contact with SSDs however and more likely to see them as stigmatising.

One Afro-Caribbean woman who did not want the police involved had previous experience of police brutality against her own mother and described herself therefore as 'no lover of the police'. However it would be wrong to assume that ethnic minority women necessarily wanted to avoid police involvement and the protection and recognition that prosecution can offer (or appear to offer). The other Afro-Caribbean woman in this study did, after initial confusion, want the police involved but the doctor whom she told did not contact them, possibly influenced by that borough's policy of not automatically involving the police in abuse cases, which had been developed partly in response to the black community's experience of police harassment.

Experience of agency involvement is discussed further in the next chapter. There were a number of ways however in which this could inhibit further help seeking. The experience of disbelief and/or blame from both informal and formal sources intensified fears of going (or staying) public. Lack of effective action (especially prosecution) undermined the legitimacy of state agencies, leaving two women talking of independent action against the abuser as the solution. Some of the women's sense of disillusion perhaps reflected unrealistic expectations of professionals, who were thought to have the power and resources to solve a problem they were unable to resolve themselves. However, the likelihood that agencies will take effective action is an important consideration for mothers in seeking help since to go public with no confidence that protection will result often means increasing the risk of violence to themselves and the child. Loss of control and the lack of validity accorded their own experience and wishes contributed further inhibitions to their ongoing contact with professionals.

The women's past experience of help and sense of identity also influenced their attitudes. Two women had past experience of social work involvement with the abused or other children and regarded it positively, as relieving them from sole responsibility. They expressed no ambivalence about seeking help, expecting to share responsibility again, although both became disillusioned at the ineffectiveness of the legal response. Several others expressed pride in never having needed help before and being used to standing on their own two feet. The assumption agencies made that they needed ongoing help or monitoring, when they had sought help for particular purposes, was therefore threatening, indicating to them that they were seen as having failed to cope.

Feelings of personal inadequacy sometimes emerged in resentment at the help others (both from informal and formal sources) attempted to offer the child. Where mothering was the women's sole source of power and identity, and they had been used to defending this against critical partners, some expressed ambivalence about the involvement of others (including schools and doctors as well as social workers) over other issues of child welfare as well as the abuse. They were both angry and unhappy at the total responsibility they held, wanting relief, and at the same time threatened by the fear that others might perform their role better than they could. This meant that mediating across the boundary between the home and the outside world became problematic in relation to their children, and battles with professionals had taken on the tone of a defence of their own (limited) sphere of influence.

While resentment sometimes focused on the helper, it could also focus on the child, who was being given or offered help to which the mother felt no sense of entitlement for herself. Very few of these women felt their own needs were legitimate. Most were used to being the giver, the helper of others, and not to being listened to for themselves. They worried about imposing on friends and agencies, and some talked of agencies being too busy and having more important things to do. Several wanted to use their experience to help others and were willing to talk about it for that purpose, but found it extremely difficult to obtain help for themselves.

Two further factors inhibiting help seeking were lack of information about sources of help and/or the unavailability of appropriate sources of help. The publicity accorded Childline meant that most women felt they would now, in similar circumstances, have known of somewhere they could phone. However, obtaining help from voluntary organisations, other than for immediate crisis needs, often involved costs (phone calls, bus fares, child-care costs and arrangements) and energy that made it problematic in the aftermath. As one woman said, 'I've been offered organisations, but you know, you get too tired to be bothered to trek around'.

AIMS AND PATTERNS – WHO, WHY AND WHEN

Despite the considerable pressures inhibiting mothers from seeking help, all except one of the women in this sample had talked to someone outside the household prior to participating in the research. They were not always the initiators of help seeking however – three of the children had told someone else first (in two cases another relative, in one a school nurse) who then involved authorities before telling the mothers. In none of these cases had the women known or suspected that the abuse was happening, although one had herself reported an earlier incident, and another herself reported a subsequent incident. This section describes the sources from which women sought help and their varied and changing aims in doing so.

Most of the women who sought help themselves approached members of their social networks, family or friends, before approaching agencies, a pattern similar to that observed in women's response to battering (Dobash and Dobash, 1979; Kelly, 1988a). Three women, however, told doctors first, where no known and trusted informal contact was available at the right time. When contact was made with professionals, the choice of first contact depended largely on the immediate circumstances, the perception of the problem and past experience of help seeking for other problems. Doctors were the most common choice. Five of the women had told doctors before any other professional (two of these only after seeking informal help) and a further one who reported to the police did so because she had discovered the abuse at night and the doctor was not available. In four of these cases, immediate circumstances seemed the overriding factor in the choice however, since two of the children were pregnant, one woman already had an appointment with the doctor for another child's problem and took the opportunity to tell about the abuse and a fourth told the hospital doctors when they asked why she had attempted suicide.

Other factors influencing the choice of doctors however were the belief that they could determine the harm to the children and/or the belief that the men who had abused them were sick and therefore needed medical/ psychiatric help. There may also have been a more generalised belief in the power of doctors to solve problems. Cornwell (1984) notes that the lengthy training of doctors and scientific status of medical knowledge gives clients expectations that they have objective solutions, whereas the knowledge base of social work is regarded as life experience and the help of social workers seen as more personal subjective advice.

Of the three women who made their first contact with agencies via the police, two had had previous contact with them, one over an earlier suspicion of abuse and one for another offence of her ex-husband's during which she had found one of the policemen friendly and helpful and hence contacted him personally on her discovery of abuse. Similarly one woman first contacted a solicitor who had advised her during an earlier plan to divorce (subsequently abandoned) and another woman contacted her social worker first, having already been in regular contact with her in relation to the child's behaviour problems. Two others sought help from professionals with an existing interest in the child – one from a health visitor, the other from a school headmistress.

While first contacts involved a range of different people, women also sought help with a range of different aims, which changed over time.

Cavanagh (1978) has suggested that battered women's help seeking follows a pattern of initial contacts within informal networks for 'supportive help' to increasing contacts with formal agencies for 'challenging help'. This pattern seemed broadly similar for the women in this study. Some however had also sought 'challenging help', to help them remove the abusive man from the household, from relatives, although none received it, before contacting agencies. Some also contacted agencies only for support and advice, having already taken the action necessary to prevent further abuse, and were taken aback by the series of child protection procedures that such an approach triggered off.

Kelly (1988a) noted a pattern similar to Cavanagh's model amongst battered women, adding that the process started when women defined the violence as abuse and wanted to end it, and that initially women wanted to talk, to have their feelings validated and to discuss ways of ending the violence but not the relationship. As discussed in Chapter 4, defining the violence as abuse is no simple matter where child sexual abuse is concerned. Hence help seeking may start at an earlier stage.

The aims with which women sought help varied according to their own stage in the processes of discovery and decision making as did the difficulties they perceived. While the distinction between supportive and challenging help is a useful theme, it runs through a wide range of aims. While suspecting abuse, women sought validation of their perceptions that something was wrong, primarily from others (friends or family) with knowledge of both the suspected abuser and the child. They sought help to interpret the child's and/or the suspected abuser's behaviour, and to evaluate the evidence and define it as abuse, 'cause for concern' or otherwise. They also sought help to obtain further evidence, for example information about the suspected abuser's past from his relatives against which to assess their suspicions or medical help to provide visible physical evidence. Two sought 'challenging help' from agencies to overcome the denials of the abuser and help them to resolve the conflict between their own perceptions and the accounts of family members, but not to remove the abuser. Two sought practical help from friends, a safe place for the child to stay, while they attempted to confirm their suspicions by confronting the abuser. Three sought validation of their discovery from friends or relatives, asking them also to hear the child's and/or abuser's account.

Once they had confirmed the abuse, there were a further range of aims in seeking help. Four women sought help to protect their children from further contact with the abusers (still in the household), not having yet decided about their own relationship with the abusers (their partners). Three women sought help to stop the abuse, not necessarily the same as separating the child and abuser, although one woman pursued both strategies simultaneously. Three women (with some overlap but not the same three) sought help to get rid of the abusive man. Again this was not necessarily the same as help to stop the abuse. PE sought help initially hoping to stop the abuse and keep the relationship with the abusive man and only after this failed sought help to get him out. None of these three women achieved the help they needed at the first attempt. All made at least two attempts to obtain 'challenging help' of this kind, both from informal sources and from doctors, which failed them before they found the help they needed. One of these women had initially given the SSD and her GP only hints of what was happening, but all three had at some point given a doctor (GP or hospital) a full account of the problem with no action being taken in consequence. Studies of women attempting to leave partners violent to themselves note similar difficulties in achieving the help they need (Gelles, 1976; McGibbon *et al.*, 1989; Hoff, 1990). The common failure of public agencies to offer practical help when asked is clearly a factor contributing to women's inability to leave men violent to themselves and their children.

Women also sought 'challenging help' from agencies to prevent further access of the abuser to the child once the abuser was out of the household. Three women sought help for the welfare of their children in the aftermath of abuse (wanting advice on the child's needs and/or a shared responsibility for looking out for problems), having already prevented further contact with the abuser. Two contacted agencies in order to prevent the men abusing others where they had no further contact with their own children. Two wanted justice, and recognition that a crime had been committed, again although the protection of the children was not an issue. Others sought advice on what to do and information on their options (primarily from solicitors), and advice on housing, financial support, divorce and access. They also sought advice on how to help the children in the aftermath.

The women's own needs for emotional support in finding out about the abuse, coming to terms with it and deciding what to do were rarely if ever expressed as an explicit aim in seeking help from agencies, although they clearly influenced their experience of agency response. Women did seek help from friends and family for themselves, primarily wanting someone to talk to, and allies in the conflict that often surrounded the discovery, 'someone on my side'. One also contacted a confidential voluntary organisation (the Samaritans) for reassurance that she was 'doing the right thing'. In the aftermath, none had sought or expected support for their own feelings from agencies either, looking rather to friends, family, new relationships and the Church if they sought help at all.

Studies of help seeking for domestic violence commonly end with separation from the abuser. This is by no means the end of the problem for many women, even if they succeed in avoiding further harassment from the abuser. Although some may experience nothing but relief at the end of the relationship, others still need to mourn its loss (Turner and Shapiro, 1986). Where child sexual abuse is involved, this may be even more the case if women have separated from the abuser at least to some extent 'for the child's sake' without feeling that it would otherwise have been their choice then, and there are the ongoing difficulties that secondary victimisation involves.

While the needs the women felt for help, outlined in this section, at certain times outweighed the inhibiting factors and thus facilitated help seeking, the influence of the inhibiting factors did not disappear altogether. Rather, the balance could tip backwards and forwards, reflected in ongoing ambivalence about the seeking and receiving of help.

INFORMAL SOURCES OF HELP

The responses of those in the women's social networks were important in a number of ways. First, negative reactions from kin and friends (both anticipated and actual) seemed to indicate (and could entail) the loss of their support, and hence of another valued relationship, if the mother acted on her suspicions or knowledge of abuse. Alternatively, they could represent further obstacles to be overcome when she went public, when she could already be dealing with considerable conflict within the family.

Second, validation from others played an important part in the discovery process and where this was not forthcoming, belief could become precarious and doubts recur. PE, for example, sought validation for her suspicions that something was wrong between her partner and her daughter from her partner's father, 'but he didn't seem to think what I was saying made any sense, so that was that'. It was another four months before she made a similar attempt again. If the woman herself remained convinced, she could become engaged in a 'battle for belief' to convince others similar in some ways to that often encountered by professionals (Campbell, 1988). The negative reactions of others could thus become a focus of further needs, for vindication of the woman's own experience and reality, a need 'to set the record straight'. Three women, all of whom felt their immediate family had not taken their anger at the child's abuse seriously, that they had been disbelieved and/or accused of overreacting, expressed this by writing to newspapers, wanting to go on television to tell their story or confronting directly individuals they encountered. This need however was not easily satisfied where the responses of those involved in the abuse and/or close relatives remained unresolved.

Third, support within their social networks was an important factor in the women's decisions to stay with or leave an abusive partner. The significance of social support in enabling mothers to separate from an abusive partner was discussed in the last chapter.

Fourth, as stated above, most of these women approached members of their social networks, family or friends, before approaching agencies. These first contacts therefore influenced further help seeking, whether by advising the women to report to agencies, by meeting or failing to meet their current need for help themselves or by allaying or increasing fears of the reactions of others.

For these reasons it is important to locate women's responses to the sexual abuse of a child in the wider context of their social networks. The range of negative responses which mothers experienced is discussed first below. Kin, friends and other sources of help are then discussed separately, since, although some of the responses from all these sources (and from professionals) were similar, the expectations women had of them and thus the impact of their responses were somewhat different as were the limitations to their help.

Negative responses

Dobash and Dobash (1979) noted that the responses of others to battered women's requests for help commonly both reflected and reinforced the sense of inviolability of marriage and women were rarely given help to challenge their husbands' authority and control. Similarly, women in the present study who sought help from relatives to challenge their partners did not receive it, although they were sometimes listened to sympathetically and/or offered temporary refuge. There was, however, a further range of negative responses experienced by the women interviewed, all of which reinforced their sense of isolation and stigma. These derive from the threat that child sexual abuse raises to people's ideas of childhood as a time and the family as a place of safety and the complex emotions it therefore arouses. They also derive from divided loyalties in kin and community networks, and from the attempts people commonly make to distance themselves from those they consider to be deviant. These responses were not necessarily experienced in relation to direct requests for help, but are important in that they represent the social context in which women respond, one of continuing conflict and denial over the scale of and the appropriate response to the problem of child sexual abuse. Negative responses took four main forms: blame, disbelief, indifference and rejection.

Blame was experienced both directly and indirectly. Direct blame – counter-accusations – included blame for allowing the child to visit the abusive relative, for being 'an unfit mother' and for dividing the family by reporting to the police. More subtly, there were a number of ways in which people indirectly implied blame with responses of an 'it couldn't happen to me' type. These included warnings not to let the authorities know of certain parenting practices (such as having the child in bed with the parents in the morning), assertions that the person concerned would have noticed earlier or acted differently herself and inappropriate advice ('I'd kill him', for instance). All these responses could exacerbate the women's feelings of guilt, isolation and anxieties about their own parenting, although at the same time they were often recognised as ways in which the person concerned was protecting themselves from their own and the mother's feelings. An acquaintance told KV that she was sure if she had been in that position she would have noticed earlier:

> And I thought, you stupid woman, because I mean I wasn't depressed that day and it was all right, but if it hadn't, I'd have come home and felt awful, 'cos you suffer enough guilt anyway. I thought you silly, silly woman, to say that, because she wouldn't of, she was trying to be clever. (KV)

Disbelief was also a common response. Two women whose partners were the abusers were disbelieved by their partner's parents (their in-laws) who accepted the abuser's denial. One of the fathers-in-law, when the abuser did eventually confess, then reportedly advised him to stay with the woman until her child was 16 so she could not have him prosecuted. A third was disbelieved by her son who was unable to accept his father's abuse of his sister as the reason that his parents had separated. Another woman was disbelieved by her cohabitee whose relatives had abused their child. Others were disbelieved both by relatives and friends primarily on the basis that 'he looks normal', and for one woman on the basis that she looked normal. It seemed to be assumed that so great an infringement of social rules (or experience of disaster) should be visibly identifiable – if 'normal' people turn out to be abusers it is no longer possible to maintain this assumption or the confinement of the problem to a deviant subgroup.

The disbelief of others is particularly distressing for women. As MG said, 'Everyone makes you feel a liar'. However it is not the only way in which abusers are protected by others and belief is not necessarily unproblematic. Several women had also experienced 'so what?' type reactions of indifference, variations of this being along the lines of 'Oh dear, never mind', 'I knew it all along' and 'I thought so but I didn't like to say'. One woman considered that there was so much child sexual abuse in her area that people were simply indifferent to it. Both disbelief and belief with no further response can serve further to isolate mothers by creating a sense that they are abnormal, overreacting if they take the abuse seriously.

The desire of others to maintain distance from deviance and a sense that other members of the family are contaminated by contact with the abuser lead sometimes to the rejection of the woman and/or her child. Several women were rejected by friends and/or family who refused to speak to them when they found out about the abuse and cut off further contact. Two women had found relatives or friends would no longer allow their children to play with the abused child and/or siblings.

Where they were not rejected themselves, some women found others' rejection of the abuser himself supportive, feeling their own anger was validated by threats to go and beat him up, for instance. Others however felt this involved a further loss of control for them and did not want their anger expressed in this way. In addition, for one woman who stayed with her husband (the abuser), such a response, involving harassment by neighbours, windows broken and so on, increased her isolation and dependence on her husband.

Clearly, social networks are by no means a reliable source of help. The negative reactions that women encountered from members of their extended family, from friends, neighbours and acquaintances often added considerably to their distress. Since these increase the costs to mothers of believing and supporting their children, it would be surprising if they were not sometimes passed on in feelings of resentment against the child.

Kin

Members of the mother's own family of origin were looked to and valued particularly for partisan support, a sense of permanence/continuity, care/love for the woman herself and a shared interest in her children. Although not always the first contact chronologically the availability and responses of such kin clearly carried primary significance in all the mothers' experiences of help.

Partisan support, 'someone on my side', was particularly important in the context of the conflict being experienced within the immediate family, the fears women had of being alone and the choices they were facing. Its presence meant both loyalty to the woman (an ally in what had sometimes become a battlefield) and sharing and validating her choice. For EJ, it was particularly important that 'I'd got my family in the background who I knew were on my side' and she had appreciated her sister saying firmly to her ex-husband, when she saw him after they had separated, 'I'm sorry but she's my sister and I won't interfere' and refusing to discuss it further. To several women, relatives who also rejected the abuser were appreciated similarly for indicating clearly whose side they were on. Relatives who simply withdrew or attempted to sit on the fence left women feeling insecure at not knowing whose side they were on. As PE said: 'I don't know how my other sister feels, 'cos she's never said, she's never commented to me, she's never said who was right, never said who was wrong – she's just sort of kept well out of it.'

The hoped-for family loyalty was not always forthcoming however, since divided loyalties spread far and wide through extended family networks. The problem of divided loyalties is commonly seen as one experienced by mothers torn between the abuser and child (Burgess *et al.*, 1978). It is also experienced by the child's siblings, and a far wider network of kin from both the mother's and the abuser's families of origin. This may be expressed in disbelief, attempts to prevent the woman reporting or in withdrawal of all support. DK's cohabitee (whose relatives had abused their child) disbelieved her, accused her of trying to ruin his family and became violent to her in response. HS's sisters attempted to prevent her pressing charges against their father, on the grounds of loyalty (despite her plea 'what about loyalty to me?'), and furthermore warned their father before the police could approach him. CL's family of origin withdrew all support from her when she stayed with her husband. These responses had implications for the abused child and siblings, who sometimes lost contact with siblings, aunts, uncles and grandparents, and for mothers who both lost valued relationships and attempted to protect the children from their losses.

A sense of permanence/continuity and of belonging somewhere was also much valued by those women whose kin supported them at a time when everything seemed to be changing. This was expressed in comments about family such as 'They're always there', 'If I need them, I'll always have them', 'You've always got your family', even where the type of support was not always what they wanted. The loss of this for women whose kin rejected them was difficult to counter even if more immediate support was found elsewhere. HS, who had felt rejected by her family from childhood but had maintained contact up until their refusal to support her over her child's abuse, was no longer prepared to accept their terms for contact (silence about the abuse) but was left with a sense of not belonging anywhere and continued distress at their estrangement, 'Deep down they're still my blood and they're still my sisters that I've known all my life.'

Love and care for the woman herself was equally valued and meant that longer-term support could be expected from relatives than friends. However, this degree of involvement sometimes had negative aspects, meaning for example that the woman had to deal with the relative's anger as well as her own, with attempts to take over or with worries about the effects of her own needs on the supporting relative. The overall reassurance provided by the feeling that 'they'll always be there' does not mean that unlimited support could be expected or asked for. Finch (1989) has noted that in all areas support between kin is by no means automatic and that procedures for asking for, offering and accepting it are in practice quite tricky to handle and subject to ongoing negotiation. While kin support can be seen as reliable in the sense of providing a safety net (to fall back on in the last resort), it is rarely appropriate as a first resort since it has to be handled carefully within the context of ongoing relationships and in order that each party retains a proper independence from the other. It should not be assumed therefore that, even where supportive kin relationships exist, they will automatically provide for women's extra needs for support when their children have been sexually abused.

A further limitation to support from parents for some women was that, either because of their stage in the life cycle or because that had always been the pattern in their family, they regarded themselves as givers of help to their parents rather than receivers. Where the former reason was the case, one woman was able to take her mind off her own problems by taking care of those of her parents. However, in the latter case it meant that ongoing contact with parents could not be seen as supportive but was rather a further source of demands. This pattern of parent–child relations is as much a part of the traditional patriarchal family as is the subordination of women to men (Gordon, 1989). The effects on children of being expected to meet their parents' needs have been noted, as have the effects on abused children's later ability as mothers to meet their own children's needs.[1] This pattern also affects the availability of help to mothers from their parents, an important source of support.

Kin also have their own ongoing relationship with the abused child and other children. One woman therefore felt able, after she had left her husband, to talk through problems and decisions relating to the children with her mother. Given that she had rarely been allowed to make decisions on her own by her husband and her confidence had been severely undermined, sharing this aspect of parenting was important. However, the interests of kin in the child also have their negative side. One woman whose child was taken into care lost the remaining contact she had had with her mother which had been maintained primarily because of the child.

Friends and neighbours

Friends were looked to for some of the same types of help as relatives. They were a source of loyalty to themselves for some women, sharing their response to the problem and making them feel less alone, and sometimes of further betrayal where they withdrew or seemed to take sides with the abuser. They were also valued for caring about the woman herself, and allowing her to talk through her feelings, including providing a 'safety valve', as one woman expressed it, for their anger. Except for one woman, however, whose close friend also had severe family problems and could therefore reciprocate, there were limits to the extent to which friends could be imposed on in this way. Some women were afraid of being seen as 'going on' too much about their own problems and of consequently losing friends if, as one put it, people started to think 'Oh here we go again' every time they saw her. This reflects both assumptions about the degree of obligation and permanence attached to friendship and the value placed on cheerful stoicism. The sense that dwelling on one's problems is morbid is also common in relation to health problems (Cornwell, 1984).

Friends were appreciated too for humour and diversion and a greater degree of detachment than kin. They provided practical help (as too did kin sometimes), including a safe place to stay temporarily for the woman and/or her child and help with child care in the aftermath. Friends were also valued for shared beliefs, especially in relation to marriage and children. KV, for instance, whose social worker was encouraging her to go out and start a new relationship very shortly after her separation, found this unhelpful since it failed to appreciate the seriousness of divorce according to her religious beliefs. Friends who shared those beliefs provided some relief from pressure to remarry. PE, whose social worker took the opposite line, suggesting that she should have no men in the house for two years, similarly sought and received backing from friends for her feeling that she needed her own life (including a relationship) alongside protecting her daughter. One consequence of telling friends was that they often responded with stories of their own abuse as children. For most women this was helpful as it reduced their isolation and in some cases allayed fears about long-term consequences if the friend herself seemed 'normal'. The other side of that coin of course was that fears about consequences could also be increased by such revelations.

Those women who had close female friends valued them particularly for the feeling of 'not being alone'. Those who did not have close female friends but described themselves as getting on better with men than women, talking of women more negatively than men and/or as competition for men, tended to be more dependent on further relationships with men for any sense of companionship. Several women, including those who did have female friends, saw male friends and/or new lovers as providing some form of protection against the abuser if they had excluded him and feared further harassment. Two women however had withdrawn from or felt inhibited with male friends, one because the child became extremely distressed with a man in the house and the other because she found the child's sexualised behaviour with men embarrassing.

Loss of trust, anxieties about confidentiality and privacy, and fear of others' reactions limited the extent to which most women involved friends at all. Furthermore, not all the women had friends they could turn to (as not all had kin). Three had been deliberately isolated from friends by their husbands. Three had seen their paid employment as their main source of social support and, for all, this had become problematic in the aftermath of the abuse. For two it was a source of guilt, one blaming herself for being out at work while the abuse took place and the other giving up work in response to intervention, attempting to prevent her child being taken into care by being available twenty-four hours a day. The third had also given up paid work in order to care for her daughter's baby.

Neighbours, unless redefined as friends,[2] were primarily a source of fear, since they could not be trusted to keep the knowledge of the abuse confidential. Most women therefore tried hard to avoid neighbours finding out for fear of triggering off further negative reactions to themselves and/or the children. One woman, who had initially told everyone in her anger and desire to 'get a name tag on him', felt it was 'the worst thing I've ever done'.

Voluntary organisations

Further informal sources of support included voluntary organisations of various kinds. Religious groups were the most commonly used, followed by telephone counselling lines. The latter were valued above all for twenty-four hour availability. They were appreciated also for listening to what the woman herself was saying and feeling, including her difficulties with the child. Much of women's contact with professionals had tended to focus exclusively on the child's needs and advice on how to meet them. While individual workers vary in the degree and quality of support they give to women, their statutory role in assessment of the mother's capacity to protect the child was an additional factor inhibiting some women from raising their own worries and fears.

Voluntary organisations run by other mothers of sexually abused children are now recognised to have an important contribution to make to intervention in child sexual abuse since contact can give hope quickly that others have survived similar crises (Craig *et al.*, 1989). None of the women in this study had received such help but two had relied heavily on a voluntary organisation run by incest survivors and indicated another benefit to such groups. Both had, while in contact with this group, considered becoming counsellors for it in the future, although neither had actually done so at the time of the interview. As well as breaking down the division between helper and helped which is firmly maintained by many professionals, the sense of future participation gave them a sense that their experience could be put to use to help someone else which in itself offered some positive meaning: 'I can't leave it, it's been too tragic . . . why just let it waste . . . if there's something I can do, I'll do it' (AN).

SUMMARY AND CONCLUSIONS

In the aftermath of child sexual abuse, the role mothers play as mediators between the family, social networks and public agencies is highly complex. There are many factors which inhibit them from seeking help and a number of different needs for different forms of help when they do. The judgements they make about when and from whom to seek help need to be understood in the context of their specific family circumstances, and expectations and previous experience of others' responses. It should not be assumed that failure to involve others indicates lack of concern about the abuse. This assumption is one of the ways in which professionals often expect standards of mothers which they do not meet themselves. In the USA, where there are mandatory reporting laws, professionals do not always adhere to them, and many tend not to report suspected abuse (Kalichman *et al.*, 1990). In the UK, social workers also do not follow procedures rigidly (Corby, 1987). Standardised rules are simply not adequate to the dilemmas raised by individual cases.

When women do seek help they do not always receive the help they need, and unsupportive responses from others play an important role in maintaining their isolation and powerlessness. Since most women seek help within their social networks first, community education to increase understanding of child sexual abuse and counter the fear of deviance it arouses could play a vital part in achieving more effective protection of children. Since those who are unsuccessful when they seek help from professionals often become fearful of trying again, improved professional training and response to mothers of sexually abused children could also facilitate their ability to seek help from public agencies quickly when they and/or their children need it.

The contacts women made with informal sources of help were important both in influencing further help-seeking behaviour and as alternative sources of support from professionals. In many areas of policy, there is increasing emphasis on informal care replacing statutory provision (DoH, 1989b). Where child abuse is concerned this is less explicitly so because of the statutory role in child protection, except in the increased emphasis the Children Act 1989 places on promoting children's upbringing by their families where possible. The wider community is seen primarily as a source of referrals to agencies, rather than as having a direct role in child protection itself. However, resource shortages in SSDs mean that women who exclude abusive partners from further contact with the child may well receive no further statutory help. The experiences of women in this study suggest that, while support from their social networks was valuable to those who received it, it is by no means a reliable resource.

Voluntary organisations, both telephone counselling lines and self-help groups, fill an important gap. With counselling lines, the anonymity of phone contact and the absence of an assessment role enable women to talk more freely about their worries, and their availability provides a lifeline for women with no other support. Self-help groups too can play a vital role, giving women the knowledge that they are not alone in their experience, and the opportunity to reciprocate help. Neither should be seen as a substitute for statutory provision and professional help however. Unless outreach work is included, they provide a service only for those women who approach them and thus are limited by all the factors inhibiting women from seeking help already discussed, as well as the cost of telephone calls and the inconvenience of attending groups. Even those who had used telephone lines extensively felt there was a limit to the length of time they could legitimately do so before worries about the needs of others being greater intervened. Statutory services therefore play a vital role in provision for mothers as well as children and the next chapter considers the women's experiences of such formal sources of help.

7 Statutory help and experience of intervention

This chapter examines the women's accounts of contact with the child protection and criminal justice systems and other state agencies. While the majority of women sought help from informal sources first, and the responses they met with have been described in the last chapter, statutory agencies also became involved in all cases but one. Not all of this 'help' or intervention was actively sought by the women. The child herself or others who found out about the abuse also reported to agencies, and where the mother herself made the first contact, she often had little control over who became involved after this. Whether they sought intervention themselves or had it imposed upon them, women approached agencies with specific goals in mind, although often with continuing ambivalence. They did not necessarily abandon either their goals or their ambivalence once the 'referral' was made but continued to negotiate with social workers over both aims and responsibilities. The social control role of statutory agencies however added to both their aims (the hope of control being exercised against the abuser) and their fears (the expectation and experience of control exercised against them).

Two themes stood out in the women's accounts of statutory intervention. First, that 'no one listens to mothers' was a recurring complaint. Second, they often expressed anger and disillusionment at the failures of agencies to provide help or to exercise authority at the appropriate time or with the appropriate person. While they wanted statutory help (and often legal action), they often contested the degree of responsibility expected of them and resented the stigma and loss of control intervention could involve, usually in the absence of any effective control exercised against the abuser. These issues entail consideration of the social control role in relation to child protection and the significance of attention to mothers' needs within this.

Once agencies with statutory duties for child protection are involved, their purpose is to secure the safety of the child and the degree to which meeting the mother's needs is seen as a route towards this is contested. The changing context of child protection work was discussed in Chapter 1. All the women in this study experienced intervention prior to the Cleveland crisis. At that time, social work with child abuse was strongly influenced by a series of inquiries all of which had criticised social workers for focusing too much on parents at the expense of attention to the child's needs. Since the Cleveland crisis, in which parents were left uninformed and isolated, there has been greater emphasis in policy on working with parents for the sake of the child. The Children Act 1989, implemented in 1991, incorporates a new emphasis on partnership between professionals and parents. Many social work practitioners now stress that building alliances with mothers of sexually abused children to enable them to support their children is preferable to receiving the children into care, and considerably more attention is being paid to mothers' own needs. At the same time however, social work intervention between parents and children continues to raise complex and controversial issues, as recurring crises over the grounds on which children are removed from home and the extent to which parents are involved in professional concerns demonstrate.

It is unlikely therefore that all the problems have been overcome. The dilemma of balancing the primacy of the child's interests with the need for work with parents for the sake of the child is an ongoing one for social work. It is not yet entirely clear how the changes introduced in the Children Act 1989 will influence practice. The idea of partnership however relates to children in need, rather than children in general, and is accompanied by a new, and perhaps higher, threshold for compulsory state intervention in family life. In the context of scarce resources, such a partnership with parents may represent increased expectations and surveillance of mothers as primary carers, as much as increased support.

Where the use of authority is concerned, the different positions of abusing and non-abusing parents are frequently not considered. Hence, for example, Dale (1989) stresses the use of 'therapeutic control' with 'sexually abusive families'. Government policy too recognises the dilemmas of care and control only in relation to the family as a unit (DoH, 1988). However, the power relations within families mean that children and women often want controls exercised to counter the abuses of the more powerful members. Social work intervention involves two-way negotiations between clients and social workers, albeit that agencies have the greater power in such interactions (Gordon, 1989).

Professional ideologies also differ over what form work with mothers should take. The dominant ideology in relation to child abuse emphasises 'child-centredness' as central to policy and practice (cf. Wattam *et al.*, 1989). Child-centredness is a concept with inherently positive connotations, but one which, like community, is open to various interpretations. The effectiveness of 'child-centred policies' which involve mothers only in terms of instructing them on how best to meet their children's needs has been questioned. A feminist perspective indicates that attention to women's own needs can benefit children as well as mothers (Lane, 1986). A social work approach to child abuse focusing on women's inadequacies as mothers may reinforce the entrapment of women with abusive men and therefore exacerbate the problems of child abuse, whereas expanding women's options for autonomy outside the family could enable them to leave, thereby benefiting both themselves and their children (Stark and Flitcraft, 1988).

In the aftermath of sexual abuse, attention to mothers' needs can benefit children in further ways. Most children want to tell their mothers. Several of the children in the present study had said little or nothing about what had happened at the time of the investigation. Some had said more later to their mothers when the pressure was less. Some had not but might well do so at later points in life. Their ability to do so in their own time depends partly on the mother coming to terms with her own feelings since children are commonly inhibited from talking by fear of their mothers' distress. One child for instance had refused to give a statement until he was promised that it would never be shown to his mother, attempting to protect her. He had later told her that he thought she had been more upset by it all than he was, yet the focus of therapeutic help had been to relieve his guilt by increasing hers ('getting it back onto [her] shoulders' as she put it).

If mothers are caused further distress by the intervention process then children will be further silenced as well in their attempts to protect them. If their distress is eased, then children are likely to benefit as well. The guilt children feel derives not only from the abuse itself but the consequences for their families – the greater the costs involved for mothers in protecting them, the greater the guilt they are likely to suffer.

Attention to their mothers' needs is not an alternative to direct work with children. However, the possibility of direct work with children depends a great deal on women both facilitating professional access to their children and encouraging their children to accept the available help. The isolation and resentment engendered by the feeling that 'no one listens to mothers' may affect the mother–child relationship and/or the mother–worker relationship which itself may affect the worker's access to the child. On the other hand, some of the women interviewed wanted more independent professional help for their children, but even where it was available were unsure how far to push when the children were ambivalent about taking it up, and uncertain about what their children's needs were in the aftermath (to forget or to talk, for special treatment or normal life). However much professional help is available for children, it is their day-to-day lives with their mothers (or other carers) which is most important in their recovery. Children raise their fears and worries at odd moments of everyday life and need a response there and then. Restoring their trust in their mothers is vital to facilitating this process, and that in turn relies on an approach geared to the empowerment of mothers. If children see their mothers treated as inadequate by professionals, their own insecurities and anger may well be increased by this further demonstration of their mothers' powerlessness.

The accounts discussed in the rest of this chapter came from women who contacted agencies in different boroughs and different periods in time. They cannot therefore be used to evaluate specific agencies' policies. Where possible, tentative connections with different policy approaches are drawn. There were two main issues on which policies differed. First, the degree to which cooperation with and support for non-abusing parents was an explicit aim of policy, as the best route towards protecting the child, varied. Second, the relationship established between police and social work agencies for child sexual abuse work also varied. One borough had a blanket policy of joint investigation, an approach which is spreading throughout the country. Another had a more flexible approach with a clear priority placed on child protection, involving the police only where this was considered to further that aim. The relationship between policy (as outlined in departmental guidelines) and practice (the personal interaction between worker and client) is anyway not a direct one. Changes in policy often take time to filter through to individual workers, and their translation into practice depends both on training and the different personal perspectives brought into practice in piecemeal fashion by individual social workers. Practice is also developed through the consideration of individual cases, and varies considerably within one borough and even within one team. Much of what the women had to say is relevant to good practice generally as much as specific policies.

THE CHILD PROTECTION SYSTEM

Since 1974, there has been a strong emphasis in the policy response to child abuse on inter-agency cooperation in the management of cases, involving the coordination of local authority social workers, NSPCC, doctors (in hospitals and general practice), health visitors and police. Other agencies, including schools and day nurseries, are often involved in particular cases. This emphasis continues in inquiry reports and government guidelines – to the extent that, as one commentator has put it, one could be forgiven for reading DoH reports and circulars as arguing that lack of coordination causes child abuse (Frost, 1990). Since local authorities have the primary responsibility for the care and protection of children at risk of abuse, women had the most contact with them, and this section therefore primarily concerns contact with local authority social workers. Contact with other professionals, solicitors, doctors and teachers is discussed separately, since although they may become involved in the child protection system, women did not perceive them as part of it.

Overall, the mothers described some negative responses from professionals similar to those discussed in the last chapter, including both blame and disbelief. Such responses could be particularly devastating given the perception of professionals as powerful arbiters of good motherhood (Ong, 1985). Some of the aspects of intervention women described positively were also similar to aspects of informal help, but for the same reason could have a different significance. In particular, women appreciated feeling someone was on their side and shared an interest in the children. Although most of the women had no sense of entitlement to help for themselves, the value accorded it when received was reflected in their accounts of contacts with others, both negative and positive. Any indication that others had recognised their own suffering and the attempts they had made to meet their children's needs were remembered gratefully. Several women referred to someone saying 'I don't know how you haven't cracked up' or something similar, with some pride in the recognition of their strengths it represented.

The DoH guidelines now identify six stages of work in cases of child abuse, although it is noted that there is overlap between them. The current stages are: i) referral and recognition, ii) immediate protection and planning the investigation, iii) investigation and initial assessment, iv) child protection conference and decision making about the need for registration, v) comprehensive assessment and planning and vi) implementation, review and, where appropriate, de-registration (DoH, 1991b). This is an expansion of the previous model involving three stages: recognition and investigation, assessment and planning, and implementation and review (DHSS, 1988). Books on social work practice describe varying frameworks, depending partly on how far the sexual abuse of children is seen to require a significantly different approach from that previously established for child abuse cases (cf. Glaser and Frosh, 1988; O'Hagan, 1989).

The discussion below is organised according to the way women experienced and described intervention, which was considerably less ordered and clear-cut than any of these models suggest. For them there were three main phases: the negotiation of discovery of the abuse between them and agencies, how the problem was then investigated and assessed, and what was done about it. These do not fit exactly with the phases of child protection work from a worker's perspective. Referrals may come from mothers and hence the negotiation of discovery may be involved then. Alternatively, if suspicion or a referral arises from elsewhere, a decision has to be taken about at what stage during investigation to involve the mother. Assessment, experienced as 'being investigated', may be part of the initial investigation phase, but is also an ongoing process, linked with planning for protection and treatment needs.

Handling discovery: mothers and agencies

First contacts between mothers and agencies – once one or the other party suspects or has evidence of abuse – involve a two-way process of negotiating discovery. Like mothers, agencies go through a process of discovery where sexual abuse is suspected or 'disclosed' and then validated through further investigation. The interaction between this and the mother's discovery took various forms for women in this study, but their experience of agency response at this stage depended largely on how far it accommodated and fitted with their own process of discovery and response.

AN, who went through a joint process of discovery with her social worker, found professional confirmation that abuse had taken place supportive, a sharing of the responsibility for interpreting the child's behaviour which had previously been incomprehensible to her, and therefore a relief. However, the abuser had already left the household and she was therefore able to take nine months coming to terms with the discovery and the professionals similarly took months and then years considering their assessment, without decisions to be made about her own relationship with her partner at the same time.

KV, who sought help to validate her suspicions, also found the SSD response helpful, in saying 'Yes, you've got cause for concern'. She contacted them anonymously first, however, in order to retain some control. Later, when she felt unable to protect the child alone any more, but had still not confronted her husband about her suspicions, let alone decided what she wanted to do, she reported officially. This time she was distressed by the expectation that she make decisions relating to prosecution (giving permission for her children to give statements) within a few days, at the same time as she was still attempting to resolve the conflicting accounts from her daughter and husband. While she had moved out of the house temporarily, her husband was phoning her regularly to deny the abuse, 'and in my mind that's what I wanted to believe. I didn't know what to believe in the end, I was so screwed up inside I didn't know what to do.' In the midst of this confusion she felt unable to respond to the police request but felt that had they come back to her later she would have given her consent. No one did so however, and she felt punished for that period of uncertainty, and that as a consequence 'I had to go through it the difficult way', that is via child protection procedures and the courts, with no backing from a criminal prosecution.

Clashes of timing between the mother's and the agency's response may contribute both to the breakdown of cooperation between the mother and agencies and ultimately to less effective protection of children. In this case, the abuser was still living in the area, with another woman and her children, and no action had been taken to prevent or deter him from further abuse. It may well be the fact that referrals in some authorities tap into a uniform set of procedures that contributes to mothers withdrawing from or resisting further contact with agencies as much as a theoretical approach to abuse that pathologises mothers.

Women who continued to discover more about the abuse through the investigation process also found this distressing and sometimes felt that the implications for them of the investigation were unappreciated. Reading statements, watching videoed interviews and sitting in on interviews could all involve absorbing new and painful information, although in retrospect it could seem helpful to know what had actually happened.

PE's attempt to get the SSD to find out about the abuse, described in the last chapter, was unsuccessful. While they had clearly been suspicious, their response had been confined to recommendations of self-control to her partner and monitoring of her and the child. Her account gives a clear illustration of the help women sometimes wanted from agencies to control their violent partners and the inadequacy of a response that focuses only on mothering in child protection work:

> And all the time they're going round this, 'has he done it', and obviously R wouldn't tell them, I couldn't say anything because I didn't want to betray her, and I thought for god's sake, you know, just do something, take her and examine her, do something. And they just didn't. . . . The SS never used to come round here, that is what I wanted basically, I wanted them to be snooping about in here so that he didn't know when they was going to turn up, and they never, they just, never see them for fortnights, weeks, then it was only me and R that had to go round and see them. To me that wasn't good enough, that wasn't what I wanted, I wanted them to keep coming in here, to frighten the life out of him. (PE)

Two women found out about the abuse only after professionals knew, having had no suspicions themselves. One was told directly and the other was refused information and treated with suspicion. Neither had felt their own feelings about the discovery were considered. The approaches made by workers to mothers, when they suspect child sexual abuse, involve balancing the possible advantages of establishing an alliance by sharing information at an early stage against fears that the mother will silence the child by her own reactions and/or attempt to protect the abuser. Such fears are undoubtedly justified. However, if such reactions are expected as normal responses to loss, and time, privacy and support allowed to work them through before the mother again sees the child, their impact may be lessened.

While there are many factors to take into account in how and at what stage approaches are made, the way in which mothers experience them should be an important one as it may well determine the possibility of further access to the child as well as the support the mother is able to provide for her. The two women in this position responded very much on the basis of their previous knowledge and experience, yet both had been faced immediately with instructions and told that they had no say in what happened. FP had known of a previous incident of abuse, and the discovery that the abuse had recurred was the 'last straw' in her marriage. Hence the investigation and prosecution of her husband which followed was in accordance with what she wanted, no further contact with him, and she established a friendly and cooperative relationship with the social worker.

CL however had not had any previous knowledge or suspicion, and finding out that her husband had already been arrested, before she had been involved, was a profound shock. The effects of her exclusion from the intervention process in which everyone had seemed to know before she did, which exacerbated her sense of loss and inhibited her from resolving her own discovery, have been described in Chapter 4. It is possible that this practice is less common today, since the Cleveland inquiry report recommended involving parents early in investigations to avoid alienating them (Secretary of State for Social Services, 1988). However, it made no distinction between non-abusing parents and abusing parents. While many professionals now advocate involving non-abusing parents first, Furniss (1991) has recently warned against assuming mothers are a 'natural ally' for the child. The point however is not that mothers are a 'natural' ally but that they are more likely to become an ally both for the child and professionals if their own process of discovery is understood and facilitated.

Being investigated

Being investigated for mothers involves both the initial investigation to establish whether sexual abuse has occurred and the ongoing process of assessment of the family as a whole to consider whether the child should be removed or not. Local authorities vary as to whether inter-agency co-operation involves a formal policy of joint investigation between police and social workers or a more informal policy for collaboration which is open to different interpretations in different cases (Peace and McMaster, 1989). There is, however, a trend towards the formalisation of joint investigation, whose advantages are seen to be twofold: avoiding repetition for the child and ensuring therapeutic input from the start. Investigation commonly involves interviews (one or more, which may or may not be videotaped or tape-recorded), a medical examination where appropriate and assessment.

Three of the women in this study had told professionals, not realising that they would then tell the police. One had told the police without expecting social workers to be involved. For all of them the involvement of others against their will or without their knowledge added to their loss of control and anxieties. One woman thought she was going to be prosecuted herself when the police became involved. Another felt that her whole family were being seen as criminals and reacted with guilt at aspects of their life that had formerly seemed normal, tearing down pictures of scantily dressed women from her eldest son's bedroom wall, for instance. Another thought that the involvement of social workers meant her children were going to be taken into care (although the abuser had already left home). Most of the women had not felt consulted or informed about what was happening. Since the Cleveland inquiry, authorities now tend towards a slower, planned response, but it is still common that referrals to either SSDs or police are passed on immediately to the other. As Glaser and Frosh (1988) argue, listening to mothers' fears at this point and explaining the purpose of procedures is a prerequisite for gaining their cooperation.

Some of the complaints mothers made – for example, of unnecessary medical examinations – were highlighted by the Cleveland inquiry and subsequent guidelines have stressed that medical examinations may be necessary only if the abuse has occurred within the last forty-eight hours and that children should not be subjected to repeated medical examinations but referred initially to a doctor with appropriate special expertise (DHSS, 1988). One further issue was the confusion that arose for two women from the weight attached to medical evidence as 'proof'. Both had reported incidents of suspected abuse but medical examinations had found no proof and no action had been taken. No other help had apparently been offered to confirm their suspicions and they were left with recurring doubts about what had happened. Many forms of abuse, such as oral–genital contact or masturbating over a child's body, leave no forensic evidence, and it is increasingly recognised by professionals that the medical examination can comprise only a small part of the investigation process. However, given the power accorded by lay people to doctors as possessors of objective, scientific truth (Cornwell, 1984), this needs careful explaining to mothers.

Another source of concern was the limited scope of the 'investigative interview' with children. Video interviews had been done with two of the children and four had been interviewed unrecorded and given their statements to the police. Two others had also been assessed in unrecorded interviews with psychiatrists, one as part of ongoing therapeutic work. The two video-taped interviews based the verbal evidence of the children on a single interview in which they had each said very little, presumably made anxious by the significance attached to this occasion and possibly also by the presence of male interviewers. In order to avoid investigative work replicating the abusive situation (with the pressure it involves on children associated with sexual matters), Frosh (1988) has argued for the exclusion of men from such work unless they are known and trusted by the child, or the child is known to have a strong positive non-sexual relationship with a man or known to trust and like men more than women. One of the children in this study had refused to talk with a man in the room but had given her statement to the policewoman when he went out.

There are improvements constantly being made in the sensitive interviewing of children. However, children also tell more when they feel safe, e.g. after the abuser has left the home, and in their own time. One woman was angry that when she told the SSD of more things the child said months after the interview, she was told nothing could be done with the evidence, since it was too late. The DoH guidance emphasises the important of minimising the number of investigative interviews or examinations of the child undertaken (DoH, 1991b). However, some authorities now record all subsequent evidence that emerges, in recognition of the complexity of telling for children and in order to prevent the first interview being used by defence counsel in court as the statement, with subsequent information used to discredit it.

Assessment of parents is generally seen as a crucial part of social work investigation in child abuse work. In practice however, many assessments are not very thorough or painstakingly constructed (Corby, 1987) and they are sometimes omitted altogether (DoH, 1988). New guidelines on assessment for social workers have been issued in an attempt to redress this gap, although these do not differentiate between abusing and non-abusing parents (DoH, 1988). They suggest for example that showing remorse and taking responsibility for the abuse are positive indicators. For women whose children have been sexually abused, allocating responsibility clearly to the abuser is likely to be a more positive sign.

Women in the present study seemed to have experienced very different approaches to assessment. One had been required to give a full history of her marriage and family relationships at the first interview, before the police investigation took place. Another had apparently not been assessed at all before the child was taken into care on a Place of Safety Order.

One woman (CL) had experienced assessment as both traumatic and unjust. This was not an assessment in the early stages of the case but after a period of some months in which the abuser (her husband) and the child had been kept apart but the woman had maintained relationships with both of them. They had been asked to attend as a family for a meeting with a hospital psychiatrist. In this meeting he had asked her to explain to her daughter what her husband had done. CL had never confirmed the abuse herself but still felt confused about what had happened. She had asked her husband repeatedly and he had denied it and asked the child once who also denied it. She was thus in the position of trying to explain to her daughter something she did not know about herself, in the presence of her husband who was the one adult who did know. She was also embarrassed at having to talk of sexual matters, about which she was shy, with a male doctor, her husband and her son. In retrospect, CL also felt that it was unfair that the subsequent court decision, that the child should be taken permanently into care, was apparently based on observation of one meeting and that she had not realised the full significance of the meeting before it.

Two related issues that emerged from accounts of assessment were the need to interview mothers alone and to state clearly the sole accountability of the perpetrator for the abuse. For the former, it was not enough simply to offer the opportunity of a private discussion. CL above said she would not have wanted to speak to the doctor alone for fear of being blamed, a fear based on experience. She had felt unable to ask to see other professionals alone for the same reason, but felt they had misunderstood this, interpreting it as choosing her husband over her child. AN had been offered the opportunity to speak alone to the psychiatrist assessing the case before a court hearing to consider her daughter's possible return home, but felt unable to take up the offer knowing that her new cohabitee would object. Later she had appreciated another psychiatrist insisting that he speak to her alone, despite her partner's objections. This is another example of the authority women sometimes wanted professionals to exert on their behalf to counter the dominance of their partners.

Social work action: a) being case conferenced

The case conference provides a forum for all professionals involved with a child and family, from different agencies, to exchange information and plan together. In recent years, central government policy has placed increasing emphasis on promoting parental attendance at case conferences, as part of the principle of partnership or participation. In addition, the Children Act 1989 gives local authorities a duty to ascertain, as far as is practicable, the child's wishes and feelings in relation to any decision taken. The Cleveland inquiry report recommended that parents should be invited to case conferences 'unless, in the view of the Chairman of the conference, their presence will preclude a full and proper consideration of the child's interests' (Secretary of State for Social Services, 1988, p. 246). The most recent guidance goes further, urging ACPCs formally to agree the principle of including parents and children in all conferences, and describing case conferences in new terms, as intended to bring together 'the family and the professionals concerned with child protection' (DoH, 1991b, p. 41). They also recognise, however, that the interests of the parents and children may conflict (in which case the child's interests are to be the priority) and that there may also be conflict between parents.

The issue of parental attendance remains controversial amongst professionals. Some fear that parents' presence may inhibit them from sharing important information about families, that they may therefore make less effective recommendations and that parents might incriminate themselves and/or find conferences threatening (Corby, 1987). Research so far suggests that parents generally want to attend (Brown, 1986; Shemmings and Thoburn, 1990) and that their attendance can have positive benefits both for them and professionals, given careful preparation. Parents can sometimes provide information not known to professionals and their presence can make professionals less likely to introduce irrelevant personal details and unsubstantiated judgements and more aware of parents' feelings and needs (Greenwich Directorate of Social Services, 1986; Shemmings and Thoburn, 1990). Where good practice and honest relationships already exist, they appear to be strengthened by parental participation. The arguments for participation are often couched in terms of civil liberties or parents' rights but it may also be in the child's interests if better social worker–parent relationships are thereby established.

Two main issues emerged from the accounts of women in the present study: first, that developing participatory working relationships clearly demands more than simply attendance at a conference and, second, that mothers' participation may be limited if their views are not heard separately from the presence of an abusing partner. The majority of the women in the present study had not been invited to case conferences, but felt that they should have been and would like to have gone, two adding that even if they had not spoken they would like to have been able to listen. The three women who had been invited were allowed to attend only the ends of conferences, to hear the decisions made, and to give their opinions. For none of them did this feel like participation. Shemmings and Thoburn (1990) also concluded that the benefits of parental attendance would be gained only if it was part of a comprehensive departmental policy of encouraging client participation. The DoH guidance now stresses that 'the involvement of children and adults in child protection conferences will not be effective unless they are fully involved from the outset in all stages of the child protection process, and unless from the time of referral there is as much openness and honesty as possible between families and professionals' (DoH, 1991b, p. 43).

The second issue concerns distinguishing between abusing and non-abusing parents. The current DoH guidance is clearly ambivalent about how far to go along this road. It argues first that it will sometimes be appropriate to work differently with each of the parents, for example if one is the alleged abuser or if there is a high level of parental conflict. (It is surely always appropriate to work differently with each parent, since they are individual women and men as well as parents. The question is exactly how differently.) Next it argues that exclusion of either parent should be kept to a minimum and gives examples which might justify exclusion. These do not include either alleged abuse or conflict between parents. Finally, it comments that adults who wish to make representations at the conference may not all wish to speak in front of each other (DoH, 1991b).

Stevenson (1989b) has suggested that one of the differences that child sexual abuse may raise from other forms of abuse in this context is the difficulty a man may have in speaking openly about sexually abusive activities in front of a group of strangers and his partner. This implies that men who sexually abuse wish to confess, if given the opportunity. A more common problem appears to be their persistent denial. The difficulties an abusing partner's denial creates for the mother's ability to resolve her own discovery process were discussed in Chapter 4. The danger may therefore be that, if both parents are present, the case conference may provide a public platform for the abuser's denial, leaving the mother further disempowered in her attempts to challenge it. Professionals appear to be more likely to blame mothers where the abuser is denying (perhaps as an alternative to confronting him themselves) (Kalichman *et al.*, 1990). The combined effect of their partner's public denial and blame from professionals may be highly destructive both to the woman and to the possibility of building an alliance between her and professionals. It may also not be unproblematic if abusers do speak openly in front of their partners. Given that women experienced the sexual abuse of a child by a partner as coercive and humiliating to themselves, the open discussion of this event in a context in which they are held equally responsible as parents may well be further humiliating and alienating.

It is not only the ability of abusers to speak openly that is an issue. One woman in the present study had felt inhibited herself from speaking in front of her partner, who was violent to her as well as her daughter. Shemmings and Thoburn (1990) indicate that professionals are also sometimes inhibited by the presence of both parents. Where there is known to be a history of domestic violence, some fear that revealing information given by the woman without the man's knowledge may put her at further risk. While it may be appropriate that parental participation includes both abusing and non-abusing parents, there is a strong case for ensuring that the views of non-abusing mothers are heard separately. The incidents described in the last section, in which women felt unable to ask to speak alone to professionals, suggest that expressed wishes are not likely to be an adequate indicator of the need for separate representation.

Other complaints were similar to those presented to the Cleveland inquiry. Some women had not been informed of case conferences being held nor informed quickly of their decisions. It is now recommended practice that parents be kept informed at all stages and have the outcome of case conferences confirmed in writing (DHSS, 1988). This is particularly crucial in sexual abuse cases where mothers are confused by the scale of disruption occurring in their lives. Some expressed uncertainty as to what they had been told in retrospect, because 'so much was going on' and 'everything happened so fast', it was difficult to remember.

Social work action: b) being registered

All areas covered by SSDs are required to keep a central register, which lists 'all the children in the area who are considered to be suffereing from or likely to suffer significant harm and for whom there is a child protection plan' (DoH, 1991b, p. 47). In the past, registers have listed both children who have been abused and those considered to be at risk of abuse. The DoH now stresses, however, that it should not be a register of children who have been abused but should list only children for whom there are currently unresolved child protection issues (and for whom there is an inter-agency protection plan) (DoH, 1991b).

This emphasis is in line with the common perception amongst the women interviewed that the register implies current risk or danger. For that reason, several women whose children had been registered contested the professional construction of 'at risk', where the child had no further contact with the abuser: 'I said to them, well why does she have to go on a register when I've already told them that these people are not going to have any contact with my children again' (DK). Some saw registration as implying they themselves were at fault for the abuse. Several women complained of the stigma and loss of confidence registration involved for them when it was not them who had abused the child, and two experienced registration as similar to a criminal conviction against them, contributing to a sense of injustice at the intervention process and exacerbating feelings of guilt:

They might as well put me in Holloway for a year, I'll do my time there. (GR)

I felt as if I had committed a crime, as if I had failed to protect my children. . . . I kept thinking to myself well what else, what could I have done, I shouldn't have made him babysit for her, I shouldn't have trusted him you know, I shouldn't have trusted anybody with my children. (DK)

Such comments indicate the need for greater clarity to be communicated to non-abusing parents as to whether the register is being used to record children who have been abused or those perceived as 'at risk', and, where the latter is the case, for clear information on how risk has been assessed. In particular, it may be useful to distinguish between whether concerns about protection arise from past 'failures' or new needs the child is thought to have in the aftermath of abuse.

Not all the women experienced registration negatively. Two attached positive meanings to it. One of these felt it gave her a sense of entitlement to help. There is some disagreement over whether the register should have a role in giving families entitlement to priority in the allocation of resources.[1] Registration appears to have served a variety of functions for professionals in the past, including showing that something has been done, ranking cases in order of seriousness, rationing resources and ensuring reviews (Corby, 1987). For clients, what help is to be made available to people whose children are registered is probably the most important question, and addressing this more systematically could help to counter the negative connotations of registration.

The second felt it gave her backing in her attempts to exclude her husband from contact with the child:

'Cos I feel, in myself I feel a bit better, 'cos if he's going to ask me if he can see them, I can always tell him they be on the danger list, without feeling that I'm telling lies, you see. (RD)

This woman was in an area where the SSD had an explicit policy of support for non-abusing parents. Her account is an example of the way in which intervention could empower women to protect their children by the use of authority against their abusive partners rather than against them. Clearly, the meaning of procedures to clients is affected by the policy context within which social workers explain them.

Social work action: c) follow-up contact

This section discusses the women's experience of social work intervention in the aftermath of investigation and decision making. The focus is on three particular aspects which are significantly different in cases of sexual abuse from other forms of child abuse. First, the attempts of social workers to combine their care and control functions have different implications for non-abusing parents than for abusing parents, and women's experiences were further affected both by power relations within the family and the losses attached to secondary victimisation. Second, women commented on the timing of help. Again, sexual abuse, with the secrecy that surrounds its occurrence and its long-term implications for children and consequently for their mothers, raises different issues from other forms of child abuse. Third, women encountered conflicting perceptions of the problem. While all definitions of child abuse are socially constructed and contested (Dingwall, 1989), the construction of sexual abuse is one particularly rife with contested areas. All these issues are affected by the dual and contradictory aims of child protection work, both to preserve family autonomy on the one hand and to protect children on the other, the latter often best achieved by helping their mothers to leave violent partners. Within this double bind, workers take varying positions, but the contradiction is reflected in the forms of social control, in the timing of intervention and in the solutions offered to women and their children.

Care/control

Ongoing social work involves combining the functions of support and monitoring (or care and control). In relation to mothers of sexually abused children, the social work task has been described as 'both to provide as much support and counselling to the mother as possible, and to monitor the success with which the mother keeps to her declared intentions' (Glaser and Frosh, 1988, p. 113), where her declared intentions are to exclude the abuser from further contact with the child.

Women's responses to the dual roles of social workers, both monitoring and supporting, varied. Of the ten women who had ongoing contact with social workers, four felt mainly positive about them, emphasising their support functions, four felt mainly negative, seeing them primarily in terms of control functions and two expressed mixed feelings. While this no doubt related partly to different personalities and practices, it also related to the circumstances of the case. All four who expressed primarily negative feelings had also been faced with choices by their social workers which they would not have made themselves, whereas the four who found their social workers supportive had either made their own decisions to separate from the abuser quickly (on the 'last straw' basis) or no such decision had been necessary. For two of the first group, the decisions concerned their continuing relationship with the child's abuser (one her son, one her husband). The other two had been threatened with losing the child (or not regaining her from temporary care) on the basis of relationships with other men.

Clearly in some circumstances instructions and/or choices are necessary. However, an over-reliance on instructions has particular dangers with women who are victimised themselves and/or faced with severe loss. Some women felt they had been treated as children and issued with apparently arbitrary rules. PE, whose social worker objected to her new relationship and threatened to take the children into care if the man moved into the house with them, compared this professional control to her ex-partner's behaviour, 'I'd lived long enough under threats, I didn't need it'. In contrast to the view sometimes expressed that battered women passively submit to their husbands, they are often used to resisting their partner's control and fighting to maintain some of their own in a variety of ways. Where agencies simply take on the role of another authority setting rules for them, rather than attempting to help them gain control of their own lives, they may not only reinforce the women's 'entrapment', but become the focus themselves of similar types of resistance strategy. Two women, both with histories of resisting violent men, described their relationships with the social workers in similar terms, focusing largely on proving themselves in order to 'beat the system' rather than on the child's welfare. For both, the absence of any other source of self-worth in their lives than their roles as mothers, made the threat social work intervention posed to themselves of overriding concern. This suggests that the empowerment model proposed by Stark and Flitcraft (1988) focusing on expanding women's options for autonomy outside the family would assist the instruction role of social workers even if it were not to replace it entirely. It further suggests that an approach to authority and control which fails to disaggregate parents in cases of sexual abuse is likely to be counterproductive.

As well as their experience of victimisation, their stage in discovering and responding to the child's abuse also affected their experience of instructions. PE expressed anger with the response of social workers when her husband was allowed out on bail and they threatened to take the child into care for this reason. She felt that they failed to take into account the fact that she had found out about the abuse six months before they did, after two years of suspicion, had done her best to prevent it recurring since then and had worked through her own feelings to the extent of knowing what she wanted. It is clearly vital if alliances are to be built between mothers and social workers to listen carefully to what mothers are saying about themselves, and that their own stage in finding out about and coming to terms with the abuse, their attempts to prevent recurrence and to seek help are considered.

Another woman illustrated the effects of instructions on the process of coming to terms with loss. CL, who had been required to keep her husband and daughter apart when she had not made a choice to separate herself, did not dispute the necessity of this instruction. Nevertheless, she had found it hard to carry out, since both the child and her husband wanted to see each other, and, given the conflict within the family and her own losses, she had ended up feeling 'like I was fighting everybody'. Her experience of intervention had not helped her to regain control of her own life, and the reliance on instructions, which she had followed, left her confused as to what she had done wrong when the child was received into care.

Where women experience intervention primarily as a process of (not always consistent) instructions, they may become unable to seek help when they, and the child, need it. AN was aware that some of the experts she had encountered were 'for the fathers' and others 'for the mothers'. The pressure she felt came from those who appeared pro-mother, where this involved taking the child's needs as the only consideration, as well as those who appeared pro-father, and, despite ongoing difficulties and ambivalence over her commitment to the child, she felt she could not 'admit defeat' to anyone.

Control is not only manifest in instructions, but is implicit in the norms on which therapeutic intervention is based. CL had been referred for joint therapy with her husband on the basis that if they could resolve their sexual relationship it might stop him abusing again. She had complied with this on the basis of doing anything to keep her daughter but therapy on such terms is unlikely to be effective without other sources of motivation, even in terms of the most limited objectives and in these circumstances is simply another form of sexual pressure. She described the experience as 'going through hell' and stopped it immediately the child was received into care on other grounds.

It is difficult to assess to what extent the lack of support some women felt offered was due to the social worker's individual approach or to their own anxieties about being monitored. Even where the social worker was regarded as supportive, women commonly kept some things back in recognition of the monitoring role, one for example telling the social worker she had not been abused herself as a child when she had and was in fact coping with painful memories brought back by her child's abuse. Two women commented on the difficulty of expressing their own anger, one for fear that she would be seen as an unfit mother, the other commenting that you could not get angry with someone who was trying to help you.

Other criticisms reflecting the monitoring function of social workers were similar to those noted in Brown's study (1986): failure to treat mothers as equals, to recognise their strengths and to inform them fully about what was going on. Several women remarked that 'they don't tell you anything'. These aspects of practice, and the pressure that monitoring of mothers' behaviour involves, may contribute to women feeling blamed as much as does the theoretical understanding social workers have of child sexual abuse. PE, who objected to the lack of action taken against her partner when she first sought help and the focus of monitoring on her both then and after, and who had felt that no one had listened to her or involved her in what was happening, said: 'They make you feel like you're . . . as bad as him, type of thing, that's the impression I got anyway.'

The control role of social workers was not always unwelcome to women. On the contrary they often wanted it used more effectively to back up their own efforts rather than turned against them. JT was particularly angry that the social workers had talked only to her about needing to protect the child from further contact with the abusers, since the abuse had occurred when the child was in her ex-husband's care. The key person influencing decisions about further contact with the abuser is usually the person with the closest relationship to him (Burgess *et al.*, 1977). In this case, that was the child's father not her mother. Similarly she was upset when the social worker said the child should not go to her cousins' home again because the boy's mother (who had not believed the allegation) thought that best. This instruction seemed to her to be presented as an attempt to keep the peace between adults rather than as clear backing for her in the child's interests. Consequently, she expressed disillusion with social workers and anger at the amount of responsibility expected of her:

> To me it seems as though they, that I have to sort it out all the time on my own, that it is all the responsibility is on me, I mean I don't mind that . . . I know your children are your responsibility, but when you don't have the authority and those in charge are, you can't do their job unless you know it. And they've got the authority which I didn't have, and that is where it sort of affects you, and you think oh god I can't you know, I can't cope. (JT)

Two of the women whose partners were the abusers were also angry at the inadequate use of control against the men. In both cases, case conferences had made recommendations to prevent further abuse while allowing the abuser to stay in the household by appealing to the man's self-control. One abuser was told to put a lock on the child's door, about which the woman (KV) remarked, 'and before he'd put a lock on that door he was in and out of the bedroom, see?' The other woman (PE) was similarly dismissive:

> They said he could remain in the house but if he felt that he was going to get violent towards R, or towards [me] then he should get up and

leave. I mean I think that's pathetic, I mean as if he's going to go 'oh yeah, I'm really going to beat them up now, I'm going to go'. (PE)

Understanding sexual abuse as analogous to an addictive form of behaviour indicates just how inadequate such instructions are. It was in the context of such limited action against abusers that women felt the focus of control and monitoring on them was unjust, and sometimes contested the degree of responsibility expected of them.

Those women who found their social workers supportive in the aftermath appreciated practical help with information and financial aid, someone to talk to about everyday worries, and someone who took an interest in the child, so that they felt less alone. Practical help was important both of itself and in building up trust in the social worker. One woman was annoyed by the continual offer of talking when nothing was done about her needs for both a washing machine (as the child was enuretic) and for money for phone bills (as her mother, her only source of support, had moved some distance away). Although several studies have noted that social workers tend to be more enthusiastic about casework (Wootton, 1959; Mayer and Timms, 1970; Corby, 1987), in the present study failures to provide material help seemed to have more to do with the very limited resources to which social workers have access than their training or preferences. All the women who needed financial aid reported social workers attempting to help, for instance by approaching charities, though not always with success.

Resource limitations and statutory duties mean that social workers rarely have the time to do therapeutic work. Corby (1987) noted that consequently the use of casework skills was often somewhat opportunistic, that is to say that, as occasions arose, social workers would use them to make a point designed to increase the client's insight into their own behaviour. He points out that it is questionable whether such an approach has a great deal of effect and it may be difficult for clients to view such approaches as helpful, particularly if they see social workers as social control figures. Two examples from the present study support this argument and suggest further that this type of approach may actually add to clients' problems. MG who had talked to her social worker of her worries about her daughter's sexualised behaviour perceived his focus on her as meaning that he thought she was 'a bit of a nutter . . . he tries making out it's all in my head, you know, I'm just doing my head in over it'.

HS had been told that her own feelings about her son's abuse, and about her own as a child, were self-destructive. Since she had been offered no help to deal with them, this simply added a further cause for self-blame:

I mean all those feelings . . . the anger, the bitterness, the loneliness, the frustration, the guilt . . . they're still there, they're still there, but, you know, I've got to overcome them because they're self-destructive aren't they? . . . Well I'm only repeating really what I was told, through sort of the odd social worker I saw, or the NSPCC worker, she said OK you feel guilty, lonely and all the rest of the things, but they're just self-destructive feelings, they're not going to get you anywhere. (HS)

When asked if this piece of advice had helped her to overcome these feelings, she replied: 'Oh no, I mean nothing's ever going to take this lot away, ever, and I knew that the minute J opened his mouth and said it's grandad.' The guilt attached to her own emotions was further increased by the advice she received in response to her husband's and eldest son's refusal to have the abuse or her feelings about it mentioned in the house. Again her own distress was seen as the problem and she was told to 'get back to a normal life, get it out of the house, if I've got the problem get it out' and advised to 'take it' to a self-help group. This curious concept of emotions as fleas, that can so straightforwardly be purged with an instant solution, resulted in further self-blame when she continued to feel the same.

Other women appreciated emotional support in the form of opportunities their social workers had given them to express their own feelings without judgement or advice, including their ambivalence towards the child, and to talk through everyday worries and past hurts that had been brought into mind by the discovery of abuse. In relation to the children, one woman appreciated the social worker visiting her at home and also talking direct to the children 'because you know someone's interested'. Another whose children were required to attend day hospital expressed resentment that 'they're only interested in the kids', feeling that if they were really interested in them they should visit her at home. Another woman, who found her social worker helpful, still felt professionals did not fully recognise her own part in the child's care and emphasised: 'You are the one who is coping with that child . . . nobody else is there to help you at night, or during the day' (AN).

Women needed help to understand their children's needs as well as directly for their own. To be useful this requires attention to both the mother's and the child's experience. MG felt the reassurance given her about the effects on the child, which had taken the form of 'Oh it's natural . . . nothing to worry about', ignored the impact on her of the child's behaviour and further indicated that the social worker did not know what he was talking about. He had apparently told her the child probably behaved inappropriately with men only when her mother was there and she therefore felt safe. This did not seem particularly likely since the child had been abused while living with her mother at an age too young to understand that her mother had not known, and would not necessarily have felt safe in her presence. Nor had it proved accurate, since she had found out that the child had behaved similarly when she was not there. AN, on the other hand, had been told that her child did not trust her because she had not protected her which, while probably true (again the child was too young to understand that her mother had not known), added to her feelings of guilt for something she could now do nothing to change. It is a difficult balance to strike to help mothers understand the response of the child in all its complexity without adding to their own guilt. Nevertheless, to do so requires a simultaneous awareness of both mother's and child's perspective, an understanding of the relationship between them and of the potential for conflict. Conflict arises almost inevitably from the fact that women are commonly in the position where they have nothing to do with the abuse from their own perspective (and thus may feel victimised by circumstances beyond their control), but nevertheless are inextricably involved in the meaning and impact of abuse for the child (raising questions about parental responsibility). This is a structural issue affecting all mothers and children, not just an exceptional circumstance which can be resolved by bringing in an extra worker (Glaser and Frosh, 1988). In each of the last two examples, the social worker appeared to have focused only on one perspective, in the first case the mother's need for reassurance and in the second the child's need for protection. The long-term needs of neither mother nor child are likely to be served by conflating their perspectives or needs.

Timing

Problems with the timing of help appeared to derive from attitudes to the privacy of the marital relationship, from resource and organisational factors and from professional priorities. Three women complained of the lack of help they had received while their abusive partners were still in the home, and in all cases SSDs had known of at least some of the problems. Maynard (1985) has noted that social workers commonly pay little attention to women's complaints of their partners' violence against themselves, focusing only on their capacity to protect the child. In these cases however the woman's capacity to protect the child was limited by the continued presence of the child's abuser and they had all sought help because they felt unable alone to protect their children from their partners. The reluctance of social workers to intervene in these cases seems likely to derive from the same source, an unwillingness to intervene in the marital relationship even when expressly asked to do so, although fears of confronting the abuser themselves and lack of systematic attention to degree of risk (Corby and Mills, 1986) may also contribute. All these women felt badly let down and this contributed to the sense of injustice attached to monitoring of them once their partners had left. As PE said: 'But it wasn't until after . . . that they started becoming very forceful and everything and it's too bloody late then, it's all over and done then . . . it was all just a bloody mess really.'

The involvement of agencies once family breakdown had occurred was not necessarily followed through with support in the aftermath, when women were on their own coping with their own feelings and the child's. Earlier research has noted that too much emphasis is sometimes placed on the investigatory machinery for child abuse and too little on what comes after (Packman and Randall, 1989). Inter-agency communication may also become an end in itself and obscure the aim that cooperation is designed to foster (La Fontaine, 1990). Several women, whose cases had been dealt with by a borough experimenting with a new approach to child sexual abuse based on joint police and social services investigation, were critical of the balance of agency effort and the lack of follow-up services once investigation was over. Furthermore, social work contact seemed to these women to stop and start according to social workers going on holidays, sick leave and training courses and changing jobs, more than in accordance with their own or the child's needs. For one woman, two changes of social worker left her feeling it was not worth trying to establish another relationship when it would probably again last only a short time. Another was left with no contact for four months while her social worker was off sick.

In two cases, no social worker had been allocated for follow-up work. In both of these, the child had been abused by a relative outside the immediate household. There were thus three possible reasons for lack of ongoing social work involvement: first, that both women were middle class and hence may not have fitted the image of social work clients; second, that the protection of the child from further abuse was not regarded as a problem; and, third, that the joint police/social work investigation took place in the area of 'the scene of the crime' in accordance with criminal investigation procedures. The third appeared to have been the explicit reason since both women had been told that no ongoing support could be provided since they were outside the catchment area of the investigating social workers. Clearly this could be overcome by referring cases on to different teams/ areas for follow-up. This had happened in another case, but was also problematic as the woman had established a positive relationship with the social worker involved in the investigation and was then allocated to a different social worker for follow-up. When the painful disclosure of personal information had been involved and some trust established during the investigation, this was unfortunate for both mother and child.

Conflicting definitions of the problem

Workers bring a range of personal and professional beliefs into their practice and some of the problems these women described derived from conflicting ideas on the nature of the problem and/or the appropriate solution, either between different professionals or between themselves and their social workers. The lack of control some women expressed made them particularly vulnerable to confusion resulting from conflicting messages from different professionals. These conflicting messages derived partly from the contradictory nature of child protection work and women's position. Two women had been encouraged either to work out their marriage or to remarry, and then told that by doing so they had chosen the man above the child. Conflicts also derived from the different values and strategies workers adopt within this overall contradiction. One woman had been told that her daughter needed to grow up in a 'normal family' and the child therefore needed to learn to accept another man in the house with her mother. Another had been told that her daughter needed to be protected from any contact with men at home.

Conflict arose between PE and her social worker both over what her daughter's needs were and over how to balance them with her own. She felt her daughter needed a normal life, which included having boyfriends as her friends at school did and men other than the abuser in the house. She was angry at the social worker's idea that R should be protected from all contact with men, arguing that they were going to make her feel more different than she already did from other children, and also wanting her own life which included a new relationship with a man and male friends:

> I said that child's got, to my way of looking at it was that she had to lead a decent life, a proper life as quick as possible. They were making her frightened of men, they was at, she's got to be scared of men, and I said well the way you're carrying on, I said you're going to make her scared of men. You're going to make her nervous of another man. The way I looked at it was the sooner she got back to proper, like the reality of living a normal everyday life, the better for everybody. There's no good you putting her away from men for two years, and then all of a sudden say right R, go out into the world and see these men. . . . I mean if anything, I thought that would be the best thing, to sort of let her know that not all men are like that, he was just, a one off thing, you know what I mean? (PE)

She also needed to share some of the responsibility for protecting the child and to trust again herself. The social workers had advised her not to leave the child alone with her new cohabitee when she went into hospital and she had concurred the first time. The second time, however, she decided to leave them together despite some anxiety, feeling that she had to be able to take that risk again.

Two women described conflicting perceptions between them and their social workers in relation to the timespan involved in the problem. MG had felt her long-term worries, that the child (now aged 6) might become promiscuous in adolescence, had been dismissed. She had been told not to worry about the future, it was too early to tell. This may have been true but it had not stopped her worrying. Rather it had left her feeling that the social worker had implied she was 'cracking up' to be thinking such things. JT had been told that her child (aged 5) should never see the abusers (her cousins) again. While she agreed and complied with this instruction, she was left wondering what exactly 'never' meant and what the implications might be for long-term family relationships and events.

Another woman's criticism of the way her daughter had been treated was based both on conflicting ideas of childhood and of the proper balance between herself and her child. RD felt her daughter, aged 12, had been treated as an adult because of her abusive experience (including pregnancy and childbirth). She wanted her to have a proper childhood and felt she should not be made an adult because of sexual knowledge which had been imposed upon her. She also resented people writing direct to the child with details of appointments, for instance, since although she realised they did this because they concerned the child's experience, she was still the one who took her daughter to appointments and felt cut out by this, 'like I'm not her mother'. Such conflicts indicate the importance of social workers being critically aware of the influence of their own values on their practice.

Social work action: d) losing children into care

Parents who are no longer caring for their children are likely to be low priority for social work attention where resources are limited. The Children Act 1989 however, places an increased emphasis on maintaining contact between parents and children in care, where this is practicable and consistent with the child's welfare (Schedule 2(15)). The present study indicated two reasons for attention to the needs of mothers in this situation in the interests of children: first, they may resume care of or contact with the child in the future, and, second, other children in the family may be affected by the loss of a sibling into care.

Four of the women in this study had children in care, one voluntarily and three on compulsory orders (including one whose son, the abuser, was in care).[2] The one mother who had placed her child in voluntary care for a while particularly appreciated recognition that she had not 'abandoned' her child, but had done her best in extremely difficult circumstances and felt this was in the child's interests as well as her own.

It is not possible to comment on how the other decisions were reached or handled since the women's accounts were more charged here than anywhere else with an unresolved sense of loss. None of these three women felt they had had any support for their own feelings about the decision to remove the child. This may be an impossible role for social workers to play given the perception of them as the cause of the problem in these circumstances but it is a need that merits attention. In the absence of alternative solutions, women's distress was either channelled into fighting the system to regain their children (although in one case this was followed by considerable ambivalence when it actually became likely that the child might return) or into dependence on the remaining child.

The latter result is illustrated by CL, who had had to cope with her son's distress at losing his sister, as well as her own at losing her daughter. She had had no help in how to tell her son and had borne the brunt of his distress alone, exacerbating the guilt which both the discovery of abuse and experience of intervention had left her with: 'See, half the time I feel that I've ruined his life by not having his sister at home.' During the intervention process she had also given up her own paid work, previously a source of pride and autonomy for her, in an attempt to keep the child by being a twenty-four-hour mother. She continued to attempt to meet her son's needs in this way which did nothing to relieve her depression and was consequently highly unlikely to benefit him. Her shame at the abuse of her daughter and her removal into care made it extremely difficult for her to seek help herself and she needed someone to approach her.

HEALTH, EDUCATION AND LEGAL SERVICES

As well as their contact with statutory social workers, women also sought help from GPs and health visitors, teachers and heads of schools, and solicitors. Most women held high expectations of GPs despite commonly having past experience of being offered tranquillisers, anti-depressants or inappropriate advice in response to their own experiences of violence. Their hopes, for emotional support for themselves and/or help in challenging the abuser, were rarely satisfied however, either because of their own anxiety about taking up time or because of the doctors' responses.[3] Burgoyne *et al.* (1987) note that many patients would like to discuss personal matters such as marital problems with their GPs but few do so – they generally use symptoms to present and may then be unable to change the course of the conversation. Two doctors who were asked to help challenge husbands suggested they came in for a chat, and did not succeed in overcoming the men's denials. Two, when asked for emotional support, offered anti-depressants and/or referred the woman to a psychiatrist. Both these responses exacerbated the feeling that nobody listened and were perceived as implying the problem was in the mother's head, or her fault. As LH commented, 'I don't need no headshrinker, he needs the head-shrinker not me'. Similarly unhelpful responses have been noted in studies of women seeking help to leave partners violent to themselves. Cultural norms of family privacy appear to override the professional socialisation to help others in distress (Hoff, 1990), and a common response in patriarchal medical practice is to define the woman herself as the problem rather than the violence against her (Stark and Flitcraft, 1983). The effect of such responses is not only not to provide the help needed but often to make matters worse.

Three women had found schools particularly helpful in sharing an interest in the children, watching for worrying behaviour in the aftermath and helping to ease the children's problems, which in turn relieved their mothers. Three had however been angry at schools' responses. One head-mistress had responded to the woman telling her of her child's abuse by his grandfather by suggesting the abuser was actually her other son or husband. The headmistress had apparently had suspicions for some time that the child had been sexually abused but said nothing, and both her silence and her contribution to a sense of spreading suspicion angered and distressed the mother intensely. Another woman was angry that the child's school had gone behind her back and called in the social worker, rather than talking directly to her, when problems arose in the aftermath of abuse. A third wanted help to prevent her ex-husband's access to their children when she moved to another area and did not want their father to find out where they lived. One school did help, telling the father that they had a duty to keep the children in class when he found out from the education authority what schools they were attending. The other school involved however refused to help in the absence of a formal custody order, and allowed him access to the children who took him home.

Solicitors were by and large seen as helpful, outlining the legal options available to women, recording their complaints fully and taking action on their behalf. One woman however was angry with her solicitor's suggestion that she divorce her husband on grounds of adultery (since no proof was available of the abuse), feeling that this made her out to be 'the bad guy'. Another felt her solicitor was too soft when she attempted to get a court order to remove her husband from the house and was put under pressure to show she wanted her marriage to work. The case resulted in interim orders for six weeks. She described this as 'six weeks of hell . . . I felt like I'd been stuck in a snare' and had received no help or further action when she complained that her husband was not complying with the order that he see a psychiatrist.

THE CRIMINAL JUSTICE SYSTEM

The many factors inhibiting women from reporting to agencies were discussed in Chapter 6. Several of these related to the possibility of prosecution: fear of the negative effects of imprisonment on the abuser, anticipation of the loss of their own livelihood if he was unable to earn, fear of violent repercussions once he came out of prison, fear that no effective action would be taken leaving them and the child more vulnerable to victimisation, fear of the effects of the legal process on the child, as well as a general sense of obligation to protect family members. This section, however, focuses on the positive meanings women attached to prosecution, since these are often omitted from debate (cf. Glaser and Spencer, 1990).

Most importantly, the possibility of prosecution gave a clear message about criminality and hence the individual accountability of the abuser. EJ, for example, felt that being told by a solicitor that she could and should prosecute her husband had helped clarify for her that the right thing to do was to leave him, even though she then decided not to involve the police for fear of the consequences. Given the systematic undermining of their own perceptions and capacities women have often undergone from the abusers, this message can be extremely important.

Prosecution also represented the possibility of justice, although its performance rarely lived up to the promise. As Scutt notes, despite the male-dominated character of the legal system,[4] ironically women associate it with 'fairness' and tend to continue to believe its ostensible aim, 'namely that it seeks to dispense justice, rather than replicating inequities, inequalities and injustices existing in the world outside' (1988, p. 515). Thirteen of the cases had been reported to the police. In four of these the women had not wanted to press charges, although in each case there were also other reasons for no prosecution to be brought. Of the other nine (including two where the women were initially ambivalent but later did want prosecution), five of the cases were dropped for lack of evidence when the abuser denied the allegation. Of the four abusers who were charged, three pleaded guilty (although two of these continued to deny the abuse elsewhere). One received a probation sentence, one was imprisoned for a month, and one who pleaded guilty to minor charges in exchange for the dropping of the five most serious charges (including two carrying maximum life sentences) received a four-year sentence of which he was likely to serve less than two.

Only one of the abusers, who against all legal advice pleaded not guilty to the last, was convicted of the crimes committed and given a substantial prison sentence, seven years, of which he would probably serve five.

Sentencing may well reinforce inequalities of class and race, and it is not intended to imply that any particular sentence represents justice in some neutral way. Of the two abusers sentenced to imprisonment, the Afro-Caribbean man received seven years (for offences over a period of several months involving vaginal rape of an 11-year-old girl) and the white man received four years (for continuous abuse of a girl aged 5 to 12, involving anal, vaginal and oral rape). Moreover, imprisonment alone undoubtedly does not reform abusers (Cowburn, 1990). Nevertheless the absence of action to constrain abusers' access to children in this way leaves that role to mothers, increasing their responsibilities for protecting children from an abuser often still living in the neighbourhood, and leaving other children vulnerable.

There were a number of other consequences too for women of involving a legal system, the response of which was felt by most to be inadequate. FP, whose husband was put on probation twice for separate incidents of abuse, felt that nobody was taking the abuse very seriously and that perhaps she had overreacted herself. Hence she modified her own evaluation of its seriousness. Several women considered other means of attempting to ensure that the abusers got their just deserts when the legal system failed them. HS wished she had not told anyone but had 'knocked hell out of him' herself, although she was also aware that such private solutions would be unsatisfactory, 'it's not really revenge I want, it's justice'. Others said they would not report similar incidents in future since it was not worth it. Two women felt particularly angry that the child had gone through an investigation for nothing, one a medical examination and the other a video interview. In both cases it could have been determined beforehand that no prosecution would be brought, one because of the abuser's age and the other because the child had already been examined by her GP who did not think penetration had taken place. Given that the video interview was conducted in a borough experimenting with new techniques of investigation, it seemed that the interests of the experiment may well have overridden the interests of the child.

Prosecution also offered a clear statement that the woman's and child's suffering were not socially sanctioned. A further consequence of the failure to prosecute then was the feeling expressed by three women that their own and/or the children's statements had been seen as 'rubbish', invalidated, since they were not enough to take action. The feeling that 'no one listens' was exacerbated in these circumstances. This was also the feeling generated by plea-bargaining. One woman and her daughter were extremely distressed and shocked by this, to find that their accounts of what had happened were of so little significance in the system of justice. Filing a lesser charge to encourage the father to plead guilty is often seen as sparing the child the trauma of giving evidence (Ryan, 1986). However, while there is some evidence that children who testify in court show higher levels of distress shortly after, the effects do not seem to be lasting (Berliner, 1991b). There is also evidence that the opportunity to testify in court can have positive therapeutic value, countering the sense of powerlessness many children feel after sexual abuse (Runyan *et al.*, 1988).

One of the women interviewed had achieved this sort of recognition from the legal system. Although her ex-husband had not been prosecuted and she had consequently fought a long and exhausting battle to refuse him access, she found the judge's comment at the end of this, that no woman or child should have to suffer such violence, extremely helpful, despite the absence of a criminal conviction: 'What gave me more comfort than anything was that acknowledgement, the verbal acknowledgement at the end, of what we'd been through. If I hadn't had that I think I'd have been agitated' (AN).

CONCLUDING REMARKS

Earlier chapters have identified similarities between the processes involved in women's responses to the sexual abuse of a child and those involved for workers in child protection. This chapter has demonstrated that such similarities do not lead to easy alliances. In their contact with agencies, women received some support and help to protect their children, but they also often felt discounted themselves and/or contested the degree of responsibility expected of them. This section suggests a way of understanding the role of social workers – the key actors in the building of alliances between professionals and mothers in these circumstances – in these kind of negative experiences. It draws on my study of social work cases of child sexual abuse (Hooper, 1990). This was a quite separate sample from the sample of women interviewed with no overlap. Nevertheless it was clear from the files that the mothers in these cases had had some similar experiences, sometimes resulting in withdrawing their cooperation.

Previous feminist criticisms of professional roles and responses have focused primarily on family dysfunction theory and the pathologising of women within it. The influence of this model on the social practices of agencies has never been self-evident, however. I have argued elsewhere that there are different constructions of motherhood in contemporary discourses on child sexual abuse – medical, child protection and judicial (Hooper, 1992). While family dysfunction theory derives from a medical discourse concerned with cause and treatment, it is the child protection discourse, concerned primarily with parental responsibility, which is more central to social workers. The responsibility accorded mothers in this discourse raises more complex issues, at least if the need for a social control role on behalf of children is accepted. Locating accountability for the abuse solely with the abuser does not resolve all issues of responsibility for child protection, which may still be contested between mothers and social workers.

The problem in this context is *how much* responsibility women are accorded for child protection, and further whether workers attempt to empower them to fulfil their responsibilities or simply blame them for failure. The policy context within which social workers operate is one in which parental care is regarded as primary, the taken for granted backdrop against which agencies intervene only in the event of failure. Within this, the sexual division of labour, in which children's welfare is women's responsibility, is also taken for granted. Hence, it is least challenging to current power structures to attribute any unmet needs which children have to mothers' failings and translate any new needs that arise into further expectations of mothers. Training informed by a feminist perspective can help to counter these tendencies and offer alternative understandings and options. However, there are also pressures to perpetuate them from the social and organisational context of child protection work which merit attention.

The responsibility placed on women whose children are sexually abused depends partly on how the problem is theorised and partly on the extent to which workers are able to meet children's needs themselves. Pithouse (1987) has argued that social workers blame clients – constructing them as a 'particular sort of person' to whom it could be expected that awful things would happen – as a way of managing 'occupational impotence'. Contra-dictory societal expectations, limited resources, low professional status, inadequate training and knowledge, the uncertainties surrounding discovery and appropriate response, inadequate legal action and the com-plexity of the interaction with children and other family members all contribute to high levels of anxiety in cases of child sexual abuse. As one social worker interviewed put it, 'My protectiveness to her is like an Aertex vest . . . total protection is a myth'.

Since mothers are the main alternative sources of child protection, it is they who bear the brunt of social workers' frustration in their talk of cases. One form this takes is judging that 'she knew' or 'she disbelieved' – despite evidence of far more complex processes involving doubt, uncertainty and ambivalence – as shorthand for 'not doing enough'. Enough however is often defined with the benefit of hindsight and incorporates expectations of mothers which social workers clearly fail to meet themselves. Another is the use of labels such as 'a collusive wife' or 'a dysfunctional family', with little meaning in themselves or relationship to the circumstances of the case, as a way of distancing the worker from the client. Such talk does not translate directly into practice, since it is counterproductive for social workers to blame mothers directly. Women confronted in the heat of a worker's anxiety with no consideration for their own feelings did not confide easily in social workers again, and social work relies on such confidence. However, such talk is likely to contribute indirectly to the sense of discounting which women experience since the complexity of their experience tends to be lost in it, and it is from such talk (and its written version, records) that workers learn the history of a case from each other. The labelling and stereotyping of women, as disbelievers for example, may also mean opportunities are missed to work with them towards resolving their own processes of response.

The less social workers are able to do for children themselves the more likely they are to attribute fault to mothers to protect themselves from their own inadequacies. At the same time, the less social workers are able to do for children themselves the more they need mothers to do. Since social workers rely on mothers to prevent children being received into care, there is an incentive to develop ever-changing expectations of mothers. Such expectations are influenced by many factors. Increased pessimism about the possibility of rehabilitating abusers means women are now often expected to separate from their partners permanently rather than temporarily. An unknown abuser can mean a woman is expected to exclude all men from the house. On the other hand a known abuser who is imprisoned removes the pressure on the woman to prove she can protect her child from him. Scarce places in children's homes and with foster parents increase the need to keep children with their mothers if at all possible. The availability of a non-resident adult sibling with whom the abused child wishes to live can remove the requirement for the mother to separate from her partner. The unavailability of an abuser – whether unknown or disappeared – may lead to a focus by workers on what is available and visible, any problems in the mother–child relationship. These ever-changing expectations may well lead to women feeling blamed or contesting the degree of responsibility expected of them.

I have focused on a way of understanding women's negative experiences of social work intervention since these may inhibit the building of alliances between social workers and mothers. The positive experiences demonstrate however that there is a space for practice aimed at empowering women to protect their children. The next chapter sets out a framework for understanding and policy which might facilitate that aim.

8   Conclusions

The situation women face when a child is sexually abused by a partner or another relative is one of formidable stressfulness and complexity. They are faced with losses for themselves, their children and others, with confusion, conflict and threat both from within the family and outside, and decisions with life-long implications. The language used in professional discourses to describe circumstances in which they do not fully meet children's needs for protection is hopelessly inadequate to represent this. The key terms – 'collusion', 'maintenance' and 'failure to protect' – are labels attached to women's roles on the basis of outcome. They say only that abuse recurred after the mother had some knowledge of it and nothing of what occurred in between. It was for this reason that the inquiry into Tyra Henry's death after a history of physical abuse did not regard the term 'failure to protect' as useful in relation to her mother, dismissing it as 'self-evident' (London Borough of Lambeth, 1987). In addition, how knowledge is imputed in relation to child sexual abuse is highly problematic. Both 'collusion' and 'maintenance' further imply consensus or agreement. Their use derives from the functionalist approach to the family as a consensual unit which has underpinned most family systems theory. The accounts of the women interviewed for this study indicated that their inability to meet all their children's needs for protection had more to do with conflict than consensus.

Language does not simply reflect reality but constructs it, providing a prism through which experience is interpreted. A practice geared towards the empowerment of mothers therefore needs a new vocabulary, one which recognises what women do do as well as what they do not, and also the external barriers they face. Such a vocabulary should include reference to the role women play in protecting or attempting to protect children from other members of their family, and the role they play in mediating or attempting to mediate between the needs and interests of the different individuals (including themselves) involved in the situation. It should recognise their role as mediators between the family and their social networks, and between the family and public agencies. It should recognise women's own victimisation – both primary and secondary – and their survival, as well as their children's.

An empowerment-based practice also needs an understanding of the cross-cutting sources of oppression which contribute to the form power relations take in specific circumstances. In Chapter 1, I offered a broad framework for the position of women as mothers, in relation to men, children and professionals. While this focused on commonalities, there are also many sources of difference between women – class, race, age, ability and sexual orientation in particular. This study was too small to address all these (all the women were able-bodied and heterosexual), and too small to address any of them in depth. However, it indicates some of the ways in which class, age and race influence women's options in these circumstances, and enables some speculation on the likely impact of other forms of oppression.

In considering separating from abusive partners, middle-class women appeared more constrained by ideas of duty in marriage and fears of the stigma of divorce than working-class women who saw their marriages more as a bargain. The experience of economic dependence on men cross-cuts class (although it is not universal) but has a different meaning in the context of different ideas about marriage, and appeared to be more dis-empowering for middle-class women. For those women with paid work, however, middle-class women with access to better paid jobs were less vulnerable to poverty on separation. In seeking help, middle-class women were more likely to fear the stigma of contact with SSDs (whose client group is above all the poor), while working-class women had stronger fears of losing their children into care. Age also has a multi-dimensional influence. Older women with a long history of economic dependence face fewer options for re-entering the labour market than younger women, making divorce more risky. Emotionally however, they may have less to lose if they have already acquired some cynicism about their marriages, or alternatively they may have more to lose from the investment of many years in the relationship. Younger women may have higher expectations of their marriages, or alternatively higher expectations of remarriage if they divorce. They may also fear a longer time ahead of caring for a distressed child, especially if the child's needs conflict with the possibility of another relationship for themselves. Women from ethnic and religious minorities may be additionally constrained in seeking help by feelings of loyalty to partners and/or communities, fears of hostility from their communities if they do go public, language difficulties and/or expectations of racism in the practice of police, courts and other agencies. It is likely that disabled women and lesbian women are also inhibited from seeking help when their children are sexually abused by fears that their parenting will be subjected to discriminatory judgements. Disabled women further face disadvantage in the labour market, increasing their economic dependence and restricting their options for leaving abusive men. They may also need care themselves and have less access to certain forms of support. For example, women with a hearing impairment may be unable to use telephone counselling lines, and women whose mobility is restricted may be unable to attend self-help groups.

Ultimately, empowerment demands not only the recognition of external barriers but an attempt to remove some of them. This requires attention to the policy framework within which women whose children are sexually abused and professionals interact, and it is to this I turn.

TOWARDS A POLICY FRAMEWORK

In Chapter 1, I suggested that the recent recognition of non-abusing parents in child protection policy (explicit and implicit) is a mixed blessing. Feminists have argued for this recognition, in the interests of both women and children, but in the current context there are dangers to it for both groups. The fact that parents were initially disaggregated only in the context of separation suggests that it was motivated as much by cost considerations – that it is cheaper if adults can be persuaded to leave – as by the welfare of women and children. The discovery of abuse by foster parents and current anxieties about residential care add further impetus to the pressure to keep children with their mothers if at all possible. At the same time, scarce resources in SSDs and rising case loads mean that mothers who do separate from an abusing partner are likely to be low priority for further help. For women it is a distinctly mixed blessing if they are recognised as a non-abusing parent only when they separate from their partners, which usually involves increased responsibilities for children and decreased access to resources. For children it is also a mixed blessing if their mother's willingness to separate reduces their access to professional help. The decisions of women in my study to separate were influenced by a variety of factors, but the abuse of the child was never the sole consideration, and rejection of an abusing partner did not in all cases indicate empathy for the child.

For recognition of the position of non-abusing parents to become a policy that is empowering for both women and children, it needs first to be extended to other aspects of child protection policy, with recognition of the power relations within which non-abusing mothers act, and, second, to be located within the context of a broader set of policies.

Child protection policy

The position of non-abusing mothers merits explicit recognition. The phrase derived from the Children Act 1989, 'those with parental responsibilities', does not distinguish between abusing and non-abusing parents, and further conceals the way in which the meaning of those responsibilities varies and changes over time. Attention to the position of non-abusing mothers could usefully be extended at a number of stages in policy:

i) Referrals

Mothers who approach agencies themselves do so with a variety of aims (and fears). Some have already secured their children's protection. Others fear that the loss of control statutory intervention involves may undermine their continuing attempts to do so. DoH guidance now recommends discussion with the referrer and other professionals before action is decided on, in order to achieve an appropriate balance between protecting the child and avoiding unnecessary intervention. The negotiation of such a decision with non-abusing mothers who initiate contact (*before* other professionals become involved) is particularly important. This would be a concrete demonstration of partnership, recognising the primacy of their role in child protection, and would help to avoid increasing the loss of control they have already experienced at the discovery of abuse and the immediate impression that 'no one listens to mothers'.

ii) Investigation

If suspicions arise from a source other than the child's mother, the decision about when to involve her in investigations is a complex one. However, the case for doing so sooner rather than later is as follows. First, the mother will know more about the child (although probably not the abuse) than professionals. Second, the majority of women do support and protect their children when they are sexually abused. They are more likely to do so if their losses are not exacerbated by exclusion from professional concerns, with the suspicion of them that that implies. Third, it is considerably more important to children that their mothers are enabled to support them where possible, than anything else professionals are likely to do.

Care needs to be taken in interpreting evidence from other sources when making this decision. It cannot be assumed, for example, that because a child thinks they have told, the mother therefore knows, since children often tell indirectly. It also cannot be assumed that if the mother knows of one incident in the past, she therefore knows of ongoing abuse, since she may well believe it has not recurred. The focus for the decision to involve mothers in investigation should anyway be more what they can do in the future, given support and resources, than what they have done or not done in the past.

When they are involved, women should be interviewed alone, with time and support for their own feelings. A clear statement of the accountability of the abuser alone for the abuse should be made. Women may need general information (both verbally and in written form) about sexual abuse – its definition, the patterns of abusive men's behaviour and of abused children's responses – in order to make sense of the specific information about their children. Workers should be aware that if the abuser is the woman's partner, he may well be violent to her as well as the child.

Where women are resistant to investigation, the Child Assessment Order, introduced in the Children Act 1989, may have an important role to play. Intended to enable assessment without removing the child from home, it is likely both to cause less distress to the child than removal via an Emergency Protection Order, and to be less threatening to the mother, holding open the possibility of cooperation when further information is obtained.

iii) Assessment

Assessment guidance should distinguish between abusing and non-abusing parents. The dominant approach to assessment in cases of child abuse focuses on the viability of the marital relationship as a key focus (Dale *et al.*, 1986). In cases of child sexual abuse by a father or father substitute, it is the mother's willingness to separate that is crucial. *Protecting Children*, the current DoH (1988) guide to assessment, suggests that showing remorse and taking responsibility for the abuse are positive indicators in parents. For non-abusing mothers, anger and a clear allocation of responsibility to the abuser are more likely to be positive.

This study suggests a number of factors of significance to assessments with women whose children have been sexually abused. First, the study of social work cases found no clear evidence that mothers who had had previous child-care problems were necessarily unwilling to protect children sexually abused by others (Hooper, 1990). The dynamics of sexual abuse itself, planned and committed in secret, and the implications of its discovery for mothers, are a quite different set of circumstances to those associated with stress-related forms of abuse, such as physical abuse or neglect. It is likely that the mother's long-term relationship with the child is of more importance than specific incidents of abuse. Second, it should not be assumed that women who have left and returned to violent partners in the past will necessarily do so again. The role of sexual abuse as the 'last straw' means that the reverse is more likely to be the case. Studies of battered women have shown that they are more likely to seek help (Bowker *et al.*, 1988) and to leave violent men (Strube, 1988) if child abuse is present than if it is not. Women who have never previously considered leaving their partners may be more likely to have difficulty deciding to do so. Third, women who report having been sexually abused themselves as children should not be assumed to be any less able to protect their children than those who do not. Rather, the broader experience of childhood (and later) attachments are more likely to be significant in their ability to come to terms with loss. Gomez-Schwartz *et al.* (1990) found no evidence that women who had been sexually abused themselves reponded any differently to a child's sexual abuse than those who had not. Moreover, the present study found that women drew on their own experiences of sexual abuse as a resource with which to understand their child's, and they could therefore have positive value.

iv) Case conferences

There is a strong case for hearing separately the views of women whose partners are alleged to have sexually abused their children as normal rather than exceptional practice. In the presence of a partner who may be violent to them as well as the child and of potentially intimidating professionals, women may be less able to reveal conflicts between them and their partners which may be highly significant for the protection of the child. This is so even where both parents are denying allegations of abuse made against the father, since the mother may be uncertain or confused as a result of her partner's denial to her, but open to change given help to overcome this. Where separate representation entails conflict over which parent attends the case conference, it could be resolved by adopting the principle that participation for the primary carer and/or non-abusing parent should take priority over the participation of the abusing and/or non-caring parent. A similar principle has been suggested in relation to child custody where formal 'equal rights' for parents often perpetuate women's disadvantage and are not necessarily reconcilable with prioritising the child's welfare (Smart, 1989).

v) Registers

DoH guidance discusses the purpose of registration only in relation to professionals (DoH, 1991b). When non-abusing mothers are informed about decisions, its meaning to them also merits attention. Many mothers experience a sense of stigma and loss of confidence at the registration of a child. This is not universal – given a policy context of aiming to support non-abusing parents to protect children, women may experience registration positively as giving entitlement to priority help and/or backing for excluding abusers. However, the negative impact could also be reduced by giving clear information about what the ongoing concerns about protection are where there is no further contact with the abuser, and whether they do imply past 'failings' or derive from new needs.

vi) The use of authority

The social control role of social workers in cases of child abuse is presented by the DoH as state versus parents as a unit (DoH, 1988). It is important to consider however against which parent it is appropriate to exercise authority. Where non-parental abuse is concerned, the parent most likely to influence the child's future protection is the one with the closest relationship to the abuser. Where a parent is the abuser, weaker members of the family sometimes want authority exerted against stronger members. If women seek help to challenge abusive men and receive only instructions for their own behaviour, they may well resist intervention in the ways they are used to resisting the control of their partners. If social workers are to establish a partnership with mothers, they need as far as possible to avoid replicating the role of the abusive man (if a dominant partner) as an authority figure, and to attempt instead to enable women to regain control of their lives.

vii) Training and education

The DoH recommends that professional training should include a balance between protecting children and supporting 'the family'. It is not at all clear however that the position of non-abusing mothers is currently systematically addressed, although some reference to 'family dynamics' is common (DoH, 1990). Training for working with mothers is essential and should attend primarily to the significance of women's responses in their children's recovery, rather than their possible contribution to the occurrence of abuse. If it is to facilitate more effective work with mothers, it needs also to further an understanding of the complexity of the processes involved in their response and the barriers women face in attempting to protect their children. Workers should be encouraged to take this complexity seriously and record it in their notes, rather than labelling mothers according to oversimplified dichotomies such as knowing/not knowing, believing/not believing.

Training should stress the importance of not blaming mothers. It should also attempt to counter the tendency to do so, by understanding its roots in the myth of uncontrollable male sexuality and in unrealistic expectations of mothers, and by fostering an awareness of the multiple influences on children's needs and alternative ways of meeting them. Mothers commonly suffer considerable guilt and self-blame without any prompting. Any indication that others blame them is likely to lead to quick withdrawal from contact with agencies. There is a danger that some current training may exacerbate unrealistic expectations of mothers by adopting an over-simplified model of 'child-centredness'. Training programmes which aim to develop child-centredness in workers by taking workers back to memories of their own childhoods may encourage child's eye idealised expectations, unless they also include attention to the complexity of mothers' position and perspectives.

Training, or education, about child sexual abuse also needs to be extended beyond professionals. Mothers themselves need guidance on caring for a child who has been sexually abused and sources of information which are available to them long term as new problems arise. They also need information on the legal system, including not only the process of prosecution but how to apply for compensation for the child from the Criminal Injuries Compensation Board. More broadly, the evidence that both children and their mothers seek help first from informal sources, primarily female friends and relatives, suggests that all adolescents and adults need information about sexual abuse and how best to respond to it. This could take the form of a public education campaign involving leaflets to all households, similar to that mounted in response to AIDS, as well as more comprehensive local initiatives. Child protection policy needs to address those who do the work of child protection, and professionals play only a small part in this.

Expanding options

For the recognition of the position of non-abusing mothers to be an empowering trend for women and children, it needs to be located in the context of a broader set of policies, directed to the expanding of options for both groups. There is a need for alternative care for children, treatment facilities for children, their mothers and abusive men, policies to lessen women's economic dependence on men and preventive policies.

First, good quality alternative care needs to be provided for children who have been abused, who want and/or it is judged need it, either short or long term. Short term, since both mothers and children experience loss at the discovery of abuse, time needs to be allowed for mismatched processes of grieving to be worked through before long-term decisions are made. A question often asked is 'How long does it take to get over?' There is no one answer to this. The question is primarily one of resources, how much support can be provided both to facilitate the process and to share in the care of children when necessary. However, it is likely that the longer the abuse has been going on without the mother's knowledge, the longer it may take her to adjust to the discovery, since it may involve reassessing a substantial period of her life. Long term not all children want to stay with their mothers, and nor are all mothers willing or able to provide the care their children need. Recognising the benefits to most children of staying with their mothers in the aftermath of sexual abuse should not become a rationale for denying children alternatives when necessary.

Second, both mothers and children need help to enable them to cope with the emotional consequences of abuse and any pre-existing issues which affect these, whether they live together or apart. A separate social worker for the child and the mother is likely to be desirable (MacLeod and Saraga, 1988). Equally important, given the sensitivity of the problem, is allowing some choice for both about the social worker allocated. Some women in my study expressed a preference for a woman social worker in these circumstances, although for others, other characteristics, such as the age of social workers and whether they had children themselves, had more influence on their preferences. The need for support cannot be assumed to be simply a matter of short-term adjustment to change. Women who protect their children from further contact with an abuser (whether intrafamilial or extrafamilial) may still have difficulty coping alone with the long-term distress that child sexual abuse can create, which often includes anger and loss of trust in the mother. One recent study of cases of child sexual abuse by family members and others found that only 9 per cent of families needed no further support after a twelve-session crisis intervention period, and concluded that the classic crisis intervention model was applicable only to a limited range of cases (Gomes-Schwartz *et al.*, 1990). Self-help groups and voluntary organisations can play an important role, but they are few and far between. To make a stronger contribution they need secure funding on a basis which recognises the sensitivity of their work and their need to offer confidentiality to those who contact them.

Third, there is the question of abusers. As is now recognised, removing abusive men instead of children from the home does not resolve the problem of what to do with them next. Without the possibility of re-constitution at some point, urging women to separate from an abusive partner is simply a cheap option, leaving all the responsibility for child protection with them. However, an understanding of sexual abuse as poten-tially an addictive form of behaviour indicates that reconstitution demands both an extensive programme of treatment first – focused directly on changing all aspects of the abuser's unacceptable sexual behaviour, and accompanied by effective legal sanctions to control the abuse and provide motivation for change – and extreme caution. Herman (1988) outlines the necessary components for a potentially successful therapeutic programme, and suggests that to stop abusive behaviour can take about three years and that even then some ongoing intervention to control recurrence is required indefinitely. The possibility of eventual reconstitution therefore depends on effective cooperation between the criminal justice system and mental health services, on the availability of extensive treatment resources for offenders and on adequate preparation of all family members for living, if all wish to do so, with someone who cannot fully be trusted again. While the appropriate form of supervision of offenders during treatment (imprisonment or probation) will vary for individual offenders, it is inappropriate and dangerous to argue against imprisonment on the basis of preventing family breakdown. Even if probation orders are accompanied by conditions of residence away from home, and the child already abused is well protected, the offender supervised in the community will have access to other children.

Fourth, there is a need for policies to lessen the economic dependence of women on men and the associated disadvantages of lone parenthood. Without this, the choice commonly offered women and children about reconstitution is a limited one, since their decisions are likely to be affected by fears of the social and economic disadvantage which permanent separation may involve. The choices of women and children are clearly interconnected in this situation although they may not be the same. It is in part women's financial dependence which inhibits children from telling their mothers of abuse by their mothers' partners. If mothers wish a continuing relationship for similar reasons, children are likely to continue to feel constrained in their own choices. In the aftermath, the guilt children experience at the abuse and the breakdown of relationships is also exacerbated by the experience of poverty, even if they and their mothers wanted the abuser to leave.

To reduce women's dependence on violent partners requires attention to their entitlements to social security, access to pre-school child-care to facilitate employment, the availability of refuge places for temporary accommodation and housing allocation policies for permanent accommodation. One current area of concern is the proposal to penalise women who do not wish their partners to be pursued for maintenance payments by the Child Support Agency to be established in 1993. While women whose ex-partners are violent are to be exempt from the penalty, the elusiveness of evidence in cases of child sexual abuse may mean women whose children have been sexually abused are not adequately protected.

Fifth, policies aimed at prevention – reducing the incidence of sexual violence – would make a major contribution to expanding the options and increasing the safety of both women and children. Such policies should focus primarily on adolescent boys, giving sex education which not only offers information but addresses issues of power and exploitation explicitly and fosters the capacity for consensual relationships. Education about sexual abuse – what it is, why it is wrong and what they can do about it – should also be part of the school curriculum for all children. This needs to go beyond the 'say no and tell' approach, which can induce guilt in children who have not said no, or said no but to no effect. Children need to learn about their bodies to gain a sense of awareness of them and autonomy in their sexuality. They also need to learn about abuse in a way which clearly locates responsibility with the abuser. Berliner and Conte's (1990) study of the process of victimisation, which is based on the accounts of children themselves, could provide a useful basis for this. It is unrealistic to allocate the task of educating children about abuse to parents (DHSS, 1988). Aside from the risk that a parent is the abuser, the evidence suggests that parents generally do not do it effectively (Finkelhor, 1986b). While schools have an important part to play, they cannot address the needs of under-5-year-olds, who are involved in an increasing number of registered cases of child sexual abuse. Increased pre-school provision is needed to facilitate detection. This would also expand the options of children and their mothers more broadly.

Clearly, such policies have extensive resource implications. Without such a context however, the aim of building partnerships between professionals and non-abusing mothers is unlikely to work. Women in my study often contested the degree of responsibility expected of them. If social workers have little sense of working within a policy context which offers children the possibility of safety, and little to offer their mothers but a place on the child protection register and increased expectations, they are likely to continue to find fault with mothers and to meet with resistance to their intervention. This is unlikely to be conducive to making children's welfare paramount.

Appendix
Brief case details of women interviewed

1) AN

Aged 36 at time of interview, white, working class. In process of divorce. No paid work currently (part-time manual work in past when married).

Abuser of child: AN's ex-husband (child's father), no longer co-resident (separated before abuse discovered).

Abused child (B): girl, aged 7, second child of two, sexually abused from age 2(?) to 5, when abuser co-resident and later on access visits. Living with foster parents (voluntary care), due to return to mother shortly.

2) BM

Aged 52 at time of interview, white, middle class. Married. No paid work currently (administrative work before marriage, stopped at birth of first child, brief period of part-time manual work in early years of marriage).

Abuser of child: BM's husband (child's father), still co-resident. Abuse stopped when defined as such by mother.

Abused child (C): girl, aged 19, second child of four, sexually abused from age? to 11, abuser co-resident. All three siblings also sexually abused by father. Continued living with both parents until left home.

3) CL

Aged 35 at time of interview, white, working class. Married. No paid work currently (skilled manual work and clerical before and during marriage, stopped after abuse of child discovered).

Abuser of child: CL's husband (child's father), still co-resident.

Abused child (D): girl, aged 8, first child of two, abused from age 4(?) to 5, abuser co-resident. Living with foster parents (on care order granted eighteen months after discovery of abuse).

4) DK

Aged 30 at time of interview, Afro-Caribbean, working class. Single. No paid work currently (clerical work in past, stopped at birth of first child).

Abuser of child: DK's ex-cohabitee's relatives (uncle and half-brother to child), no contact since discovery of abuse.

Abused child (E): girl, aged 10, second child of four, sexually abused on two separate occasions, aged 5 and 8. Still living with mother.

5) EJ

Aged 50 at time of interview, white, middle class. Married. Professional occupation (retrained after ten years out of paid work from birth of first child).

Abuser of child: EJ's ex-husband (child's father), separated one year after abuse discovered, and divorced.

Abused child (F): girl, aged 27, first child of four, sexually abused from age 12 to 15, when abuser co-resident. Continued living with mother until left home.

6) FP

Aged 55 at time of interview, white, working class. In process of divorce. No paid work currently (homework in past while married).

Abuser of child: FP's ex-husband (child's father), separated temporarily immediately after first discovery of abuse, permanently seven years later, shortly after discovery of recurrence.

Abused child (G): girl, aged 15, third child of three, sexually abused at age 7, then again from 9 to 14, when abuser co-resident. Still living with mother.

7) GR

Aged 33 at time of interview, white, working class. Married (but husband currently in prison). No paid work currently (none since birth of first child).

Abuser of child: GR's son (child's half-brother), living with relatives on care order.

Abused child (H): girl, aged 3, third child of three, sexually abused from age 2 to 3, abuser co-resident. Still living with mother.

8) HS

Aged 38 at time of interview, white, middle class. Married. Clerical occupation.

Abuser of child: HS's father (child's grandfather), no contact since abuse discovered.

Abused child (J): boy, aged 11, second child of two, sexually abused from age 5 to 9, on visits to abuser's house. Still living with mother.

9) JT

Aged 27 at time of interview, white, middle class. Cohabiting. No paid work currently (clerical work in past, stopped at birth of child).

Abuser of child: JT's ex-husband's relatives (cousins to child), no contact since abuse discovered.

Abused child (K): girl, aged 5, only child, sexually abused on two separate occasions, aged 4 to 5, on visits to abusers' house. Still living with mother.

10) KV

Aged 32 at time of interview, white, working class. In process of divorce. No paid work currently (clerical work before marriage, stopped at birth of first child).

Abuser of child: KV's ex-husband (child's father), separated shortly after abuse confirmed.

Abused child (L): girl, aged 13, first of two, sexually abused from age 8 to 12, when abuser co-resident. Still living with mother.

11) LH

Aged 49 at time of interview, white, working class. Cohabiting. Part-time manual work currently (and throughout most of marriage).

Abuser of child: LH's ex-husband (child's father), separated after about five years of suspicion. Abuser still living with 'child', now aged 26.

Abused child (M): girl, aged 26, second of four, sexually abused from age 13(?), ongoing, abuser co-resident. Living with father.

12) MG

Aged 22 at time of interview, white, working class. Divorced. No paid work currently, but planning part-time manual work.

Abuser of child: MG's ex-husband (child's stepfather), separated before abuse discovered.

Abused child (N): girl, aged 6, first of three, sexually abused from age 2 to 5, when abuser co-resident, and later on access visits. Still living with mother.

13) NF

Aged 39 at time of interview, white, working class. Married. No paid work currently (part-time manual work before married, stopped at birth of first child).

Abuser of child: NF's ex-cohabitee (not child's father), separated shortly after abuse discovered.

Abused child (P): girl, aged 6, third of three, sexually abused aged 5 over period of months when abuser co-resident. Living with foster parents (on permanent care order).

14) PE

Aged 35 at time of interview, white, working class. Cohabiting. Clerical work currently (and throughout most of prior cohabiting relationship).

Abuser of child: PE's ex-cohabitee (not child's father), separated six months after abuse confirmed.

Abused child (R): girl, aged 13, only child, sexually abused from age 5 to 12, when abuser co-resident. Still living with mother.

15) RD

Aged 35 at time of interview, Afro-Caribbean, working class. In process of divorce. No paid work currently, but planning part-time manual work.

Abuser of child: RD's ex-husband (stepfather to child), separated shortly after abuse discovered.

Abused child (S): girl, aged 13, first of three, sexually abused from age 11 to 12, when abuser co-resident. Still living with mother.

Notes

1 CHILD SEXUAL ABUSE AND MOTHERS: THE ISSUES

1 See Hooper (1992) for a fuller discussion of historical trends in incidence and definition.
2 The role that mothers may play in protecting a child from their partners' abuse is recognised only in its absence. 'Failure to protect' is regarded as a form of abuse (Jones *et al.*, 1987) and is a label attached primarily to women.
3 Prevalence rates depend crucially on the definition of abuse used. This study used nine different definitions offering prevalence rates for each. The figures given in the text relate to the broadest definition of abuse. Using a narrower definition, excluding non-contact abuse and lowering the age cut-off point to 16, 27 per cent of young women and 11 per cent of young men reported abuse.
4 Other findings include 69 per cent of mothers being supportive in a study of abuse by family members and others (de Jong, 1988); 47 per cent of mothers somewhat or very protective and 58 per cent having nurturing relationships with their children in a study of abuse by family members and others (Faller, 1988b); 78 per cent of mothers believing abuse had taken place in a study of sexual abuse by family members (Sirles and Franke, 1989); 66.7 per cent of mothers believing abuse by fathers/father substitutes (Sirles and Lofberg, 1990); 76 per cent of mothers being supportive in a sample of children sexually abused by family members (Everson *et al.*, 1989); 74 per cent of mothers either totally or largely believing in a sample including intrafamilial and extrafamilial abuse (Pellegrin and Wagner, 1990); approximately 70 per cent of mothers believing and supporting their children in two studies cited by Jones (1991).
5 The children and related inquiries were Jasmine Beckford (London Borough of Brent, 1985), Tyra Henry (London Borough of Lambeth, 1987) and Kimberley Carlile (London Borough of Greenwich, 1987).
6 The story of the Cleveland crisis is told in Campbell (1988), and further analysed in La Fontaine (1990) and Parton (1991). For the inquiry report, see Secretary of State for Social Services (1988).
7 The inquiries into the deaths of both Kimberley Carlile and Tyra Henry noted that the mothers were themselves battered by the men concerned. The link between violence against women and the abuse of their children, both physical (Stark and Flitcraft, 1988; Bowker *et al.*, 1988) and sexual (Truesdell *et al.*, 1986), is well-established by research.

8 Maria Colwell was battered to death by her stepfather, after being returned home to her natural mother, against her expressed wishes.

9 See Baghramian and Kershaw (1989), Wright and Portnoy (1990) and Brodie and Weighell (1990).

10 The Criminal Justice Act 1988 abolished the corroboration requirement for unsworn evidence and made allowance for children to give evidence in the Crown Court through a live, closed-circuit television link. The Pigot Committee (1989) suggested a number of further changes, including arrangements for children to give evidence before the trial (and be recorded on videotape) and to be cross-examined in an informal hearing (again recorded on videotape), to avoid the distress currently caused by long delays and by appearance in court. At the time of writing, these recommendations have been only partially accepted. The Criminal Justice Act 1991 allows for an initial interview with children to be recorded out of court and for the videotape to be used as evidence, but still requires children to attend the trial for cross-examination.

11 I have used the language of custody and access here since at the time of writing these are the contexts in which this myth has arisen, and to which the relevant research relates.

12 See also Corwin *et al.* (1987) and Berliner (1991a) for discussion of this issue.

2 THE STUDY: AIMS AND METHODS

1 See Abbott and Sapsford (1987), Abbott (1987), Erikson and Goldthorpe (1988) and Leiulfsrud and Woodward (1988) for debates on this.

2 See Kelly (1988a) for a similar practice.

3 LOSS: THE MEANING OF CHILD SEXUAL ABUSE TO MOTHERS

1 Two studies of middle-class mothers have highlighted this variability. Raphael-Leff (1983) suggests two basic models of mothering: the 'regulator' in which the mother expects the baby to adapt to her and the 'facilitator' in which the mother adapts to the baby. Ribbens (1990) identifies three approaches to child-rearing, 'directive', 'adaptive' and 'negotiative', linked to different ways of making sense of children, as 'little devils', 'innocent angels' and 'small people'. She suggests these are typifications on which women may draw in different ways, rather than fixed groups.

2 Rape in marriage was made a criminal offence in Scotland in 1989. While a similar change was under review by the Law Commission in England and Wales, the Court of Appeal ruled that husbands' immunity to conviction for rape was anachronistic and offensive and removed it. Such a change has important symbolic significance and some substantive significance. Convictions have now been achieved. However, given the phallocentric discourse within which rape trials are conducted (Smart, 1989), convictions are likely to remain difficult.

3 See Metropolitan Police and Bexley Social Services (1987) and Secretary of State for Social Services (1988), for accounts of this problem in training.

4 Egeland *et al.* (1988) found that all forms of childhood abuse and neglect were less likely to have a negative impact on mothering in adult life where women had received emotional support from a non-abusive adult during childhood, participated in therapy at some point in their lives or had a non-abusive, stable and satisfying relationship with an adult partner. It is likely that other forms of relationship, which are intimate, stable and non-abusive, also have such reparative potential.

4 FINDING OUT: THE DISCOVERY PROCESS

1 Definitions vary across a number of parameters: the cut-off point of childhood (18 or younger), the relationship of the perpetrator to the child (intrafamilial and/or extrafamilial), the age difference between victim and perpetrator (commonly a five-year age gap or more defines the activity as abuse), and the type of sexual activity (especially whether or not activities not involving physical contact are included) (Wyatt and Powell, 1988).
2 In focusing only on the power derived from age difference, however, there is a danger of masking abuse by peers. While the problems of defining abuse by peers remain not fully resolved, Kelly *et al.* (1991) took young people's own definitions of their childhood experiences as their starting point, and found over a quarter of the abuse their respondents reported was abuse by peers.
3 Myer (1984) found that the angrier women were towards the perpetrators, the more likely they were to protect their children and engage in treatment.

5 WORKING IT OUT: THE CONTEXT AND PROCESS OF RESPONSE

1 Such a stereotype was evident in the response of social workers to the Tyra Henry case, and appears to have resulted in unreasonable expectations of what the maternal grandmother would be able to cope with (Channer and Parton, 1990).
2 See Pahl (1989) for discussion of the different patterns of control over resources within households.
3 There are similarities with the situation of women with unwanted pregnancies. The failure to use effective contraception has often been attributed to psychological conflicts about pregnancy. Luker (1975) suggests however that it is the product of 'taking chances' in the context of the costs and benefits of contraception and pregnancy as perceived at the time of intercourse.

6 HELP-SEEKING DECISIONS AND EXPERIENCE OF INFORMAL HELP

1 See, for example, Courtois & Sprei (1988) for discussion of 'parentification' on sexually abused children.
2 See Willmott (1986) for the difficulties of differentiating between the roles of friend and neighbour, and the importance of recognising as 'local friends' those who are sometimes categorised as neighbours. In the present study, the women's own definitions were followed.

7 STATUTORY HELP AND EXPERIENCE OF INTERVENTION

1 Corby (1987) takes it for granted that the register should not have a role in giving families entitlement to priority in the allocation of resources. Brown (1986) in contrast assumes that it does. In the past the DoH guidelines (DHSS, 1988; DoH, 1991) have not addressed this issue. The most recent guidance however states that registration 'should not be used to obtain resources which might otherwise not be available to the family' (DoH, 1991b, p. 48), a form of words which is open to various interpretations.

2 Voluntary care is replaced under the Children Act 1989 by the concept of 'accommodation' in an attempt to reduce its stigma. I have used the old term as this was the framework which existed at the period to which the study refers.

3 Kirkwood's (1991) study of formerly abused women in the UK and USA highlights the cultural specificity of such expectations. Women in the USA had only sought medical help if absolutely necessary for extreme physical injury or illness. They did not share the expectations of women in the UK that doctors address emotional issues as well.

4 For example, the view that husbands have undisputed rights over their wives' sexuality is commonly reflected in the mitigating factors used in cases of father–daughter incest. A study of sentencing practice found that breakdown in sexual relations between husband and wife led to reduction of sentence in over 80 per cent of cases (Mitra, 1987).

Bibliography

Abbott, P. (1987) 'Women's social class identification: does husband's occupation make a difference?', *Sociology*, 21, 1: 91–103.

Abbott, P. and Sapsford, R. (1987) *Women and Social Class*, London: Tavistock.

Backett, K. (1982) *Mothers and Fathers: A Study of the Development and Negotiation of Parental Behaviour*, London: Macmillan.

Baetz, R. (1984) 'The coming-out process: violence vs lesbians', in T. Darty and S. Potter (eds), *Women-Identified Women*, Palo Alto, California: Mayfield.

Baghramian, A. and Kershaw, S. (1989) 'Child sexual abuse: we are all survivors like our children', *Social Work Today*, 10.8.89, 20–1.

Baker Miller, J. (1988) *Towards a New Psychology of Women*, London: Penguin, 2nd edn.

Barron, J. (1990) *Not Worth the Paper . . . ? The Effectiveness of Legal Protection for Women and Children Experiencing Domestic Violence*, Bristol: WAFE.

Bender, L. and Blau, A. (1937) 'The reaction of children to sexual relationships with adults', *American Journal of Orthopsychiatry*, 7: 500–18.

Bentovim, A., Elton, A. and Tranter, M. (1987) 'Prognosis for rehabilitation after abuse', *Adoption and Fostering*, 11, 1: 26–31.

Berger, P.L. and Luckman, T. (1967) *The Social Construction of Reality*, Harmondsworth: Penguin.

Berliner, L. (1991a) 'Interviewing families', in K. Murray and D. Gough (eds), *Intervening in Child Sexual Abuse*, Edinburgh: Scottish Academic Press.

Berliner, L. (1991b) 'Treating the effects of sexual assault', in K. Murray and D. Gough (eds), *Intervening in Child Sexual Abuse*, Edinburgh: Scottish Academic Press.

Berliner, L. and Conte, J.R. (1990) 'The process of victimisation: the victims' perspective', *Child Abuse and Neglect*, 14: 29–40.

Berliner, L. and Wheeler, J.R. (1987) 'Treating the effects of sexual abuse in children', *Journal of Interpersonal Violence*, 2, 4: 415–34.

Bograd, M. (1988a) 'Feminist perspectives on wife abuse: an introduction', in K. Yllo and M. Bograd (eds), *Feminist Perspectives on Wife Abuse*, London: Sage.

Bograd, M. (1988b) 'How battered women and abusive men account for domestic violence: excuses, justifications or explanations?', in G.T. Hotaling *et al.* (eds), *Coping with Family Violence: Research and Policy Perspectives*, London: Sage.

Boulton, M.G. (1983) *On Being a Mother: A Study of Women with Pre-school Children*, London: Tavistock.

Boushel, M. and Noakes, S. (1988) 'Islington Social Services: developing a policy on child sexual abuse', *Feminist Review*, 28: 150–7.

Bowker, L.H., Barbittel, M. and McFerrow, J.R. (1988) 'On the relationship between wife beating and child abuse', in K. Yllo and M. Bograd (eds), *Feminist Perspectives on Wife Abuse*, London: Sage.

Brannen, J. and Collard, J. (1982) *Marriages in Trouble: The Process of Seeking Help*, London: Tavistock.

Breakwell, G. (1986) *Coping with Threatened Identities*, London: Methuen.

Brodie, H. and Weighell, P. (1990) 'Picking up the pieces', *Social Work Today*, 15.2.90, 20–1.

Broussard, S.D. and Wagner, W.G. (1988) 'Child sexual abuse: who is to blame?', *Child Abuse and Neglect*, 12: 563–9.

Brown, C. (1986) *Child Abuse Parents Speaking: Parents' Impressions of Social Workers and the Social Work Process*, Working Paper 63, SAUS, University of Bristol.

Brown, G. and Harris, T. (1978) *Social Origins of Depression*, London: Tavistock.

Burgess, A.W., Holstrom, L.L. and McCausland, M.P. (1977) 'Child sexual assault by a family member: decisions following disclosure', *Victimology: An International Journal*, II, 2: 236–50.

Burgess, A.W., Holstrom, L.L. and McCausland, M.P. (1978) 'Divided loyalty in incest cases', in A.W. Burgess *et al.*, *Sexual Assault of Children and Adolescents*, Lexington, Mass.: Lexington Books.

Burgess, R.L. and Youngblade, L.M. (1988) 'Social incompetence and the intergenerational transmission of abusive parental practices', in G.T. Hotaling *et al.* (eds), *Family Abuse and its Consequences: New Directions in Research*, London: Sage.

Burgoyne, J., Ormrod, R. and Richards, M. (1987) *Divorce Matters*, Harmondsworth: Penguin.

Cammaert, L.A. (1988) 'Nonoffending mothers: a new conceptualisation', in L. Walker (ed.), *Handbook on Sexual Abuse of Children*, New York: Springer.

Campbell, B. (1988) *Unofficial Secrets: Child Sexual Abuse – The Cleveland Case*, London: Virago.

Caplan, P.J. (1990) 'Making mother-blaming visible: the emperor's new clothes', *Women and Therapy*, 10, 1/2: 61–70.

Cavanagh, C. (1978) *Battered Women and Social Control*, University of Stirling: MA Thesis.

Channer, Y. and Parton, N. (1990) 'Racism, cultural relativism and child protection', in The Violence Against Children Study Group, *Taking Child Abuse Seriously*, London: Unwin Hyman.

Chodorow, N. and Contratto, S. (1982) 'The fantasy of the perfect mother', in B. Thorne and M. Yalom (eds), *Rethinking the Family: Some Feminist Questions*, New York: Longman.

Cohen, B. (1990) *Caring for Children: the 1990 Report*, London: Family Policy Studies Centre.

Cohen, G. (1977) 'Absentee husbands in spiralist families', *Journal of Marriage and the Family*, 39: 595–604.

Conte, J.R. and Berliner, L. (1988) 'The impact of sexual abuse on children: empirical findings', in L. Walker (ed.), *Handbook on Sexual Abuse of Children*, New York: Springer.

Conte, J., Wolf, S. and Smith, T. (1989) 'What sexual offenders tell us about prevention: preliminary findings', *Child Abuse and Neglect*, 13: 293–301.

Cooper, D.M. and Ball, D. (1987) *Social Work and Child Abuse*, London: Macmillan Education.

Corby, B. (1987) *Working with Child Abuse: Social Work Practice and the Child Abuse System*, Milton Keynes: Open University Press.

Corby, B. and Mills, C. (1986) 'Child abuse: risks and resources', *British Journal of Social Work*, 16: 531–42.

Cornwell, J. (1984) *Hard-Earned Lives: Accounts of Health and Illness from East London*, London: Tavistock.

Corwin, D.L. *et al.* (1987) 'Child sexual abuse and custody disputes', *Journal of Interpersonal Violence*, 2, 1: 91–105.

Courtois, C. and Sprei, J. (1988) 'Retrospective incest therapy for women', in L. Walker (ed.), *Handbook on Sexual Abuse of Children*, New York: Springer.

Cowburn, M. (1990) 'Work with sexual offenders in prisons: what happens to nonces?'. Paper presented at Conference on Child Sexual Abuse: Research and Policy Issues, Institute of Child Health, 19/20.3.90.

Craig, E., Erooga, M., Morrison, T. and Shearer, E. (1989) 'Making sense of sexual abuse – charting the sifting sands', in C. Wattam *et al.* (eds), *Child Sexual Abuse*, Harlow: Longman.

Dale, P. (1989) 'Management implications of child sexual abuse', in P. Sills (ed.), *Child Abuse: Challenges for Policy and Practice*, Wallington: Community Care/Reed Business Publishing.

Dale, P., Davies, M., Morrison, T. and Waters, J. (1986) *Dangerous Families: Assessment and Treatment of Child Abuse*, London: Tavistock.

de Francis, V. (1969) *Protecting the Child Victim of Sex Crimes Committed by Adults, Final Report*, Denver, Colorado: American Humane Association.

de Jong, A.R. (1986) 'Childhood sexual abuse precipitating maternal hospitalisation', *Child Abuse and Neglect*, 10: 551–3.

de Jong, A.R. (1988) 'Maternal responses to the sexual abuse of their children', *Pediatrics*, 81, 1: 14–21.

Delphy, C. (1984) *Close to Home: A Materialist Analysis of Women's Oppression*, London: Hutchinson.

Dempster, H.L. (1989) 'The Reactions and Responses of Women to the Sexual Abuse of their Children: A Feminist View and Analysis'. Unpublished MSc dissertation, Dept of Sociology and Social Policy, University of Stirling.

Department of Health and Social Security (1985) *Social Work Decisions in Child Care: Recent Research Findings and their Implications*, London: HMSO.

Department of Health and Social Security (1988) *Working Together: A Guide to Arrangements for Inter-Agency Cooperation for the Protection of Children from Abuse*, London: HMSO.

Department of Health (1988) *Protecting Children: A Guide for Social Workers Undertaking a Comprehensive Assessment*, London: HMSO.

Department of Health (1989a) *Working with Child Sexual Abuse: Guidelines for Training Social Services Staff*, Training Support Programme (Child Care).

Department of Health (1989b) *Caring for People: Community Care in the Next Decade and Beyond*, London: HMSO.

Department of Health (1990) *Working with Child Sexual Abuse: A Review of the Impact of Training Guidelines*, London: SSI.

Department of Health (1991a) *Working Together: A Guide to Arrangements for Inter-Agency Cooperation for the Protection of Children from Abuse (Guidance)* (Consultation Paper Number 22).

Department of Health (1991b) *Working Together Under the Children Act 1989*, London: HMSO.

Dietz, C.A. and Craft, J.L. (1980) 'Family dynamics of incest: a new perspective', *Social Casework*, December: 602–9.

Dingwall, R. (1989) 'Some problems about predicting child abuse and neglect', in O. Stevenson (ed.), *Child Abuse: Public Policy and Professional Practice*, Hemel Hempstead: Harvester Wheatsheaf.

DiSabatino, J. (1989) 'Protect the child, neglect her family', *Child Abuse Review*, 3, 1: 16–18.

Dobash, R.E. and Dobash, R.P. (1979) *Violence against Wives: A Case against the Patriarchy*, New York: The Free Press.

Driver, E. and Droisen, A. (eds) (1989) *Child Sexual Abuse: Feminist Perspectives*, London: Macmillan Education.

Egeland, B., Jacobvitz, D. and Stroufe, L.A. (1988) 'Breaking the cycle of abuse', *Child Development*, 59: 1080–8.

Eichler, M. (1988) *Non-Sexist Research Methods: A Practical Guide*, Boston: Allen and Unwin.

Eisenberg, N., Owens, R.C. and Dewey, M.E. (1987) 'Attitudes of health professionals to child sexual abuse and incest', *Child Abuse and Neglect*, 11, 1: 109–16.

Elton, A. (1988) 'Assessment of families for treatment', in A Bentovim *et al.* (eds), *Child Sexual Abuse within the Family*, London: Wright.

Ennew, J. (1986) *The Sexual Exploitation of Children*, Cambridge: Polity.

Erikson, R. and Goldthorpe, J.H. (1988) 'Women at class crossroads: a critical note', *Sociology*, 22, 4: 545–53.

Everson, M.D., Hunter, W.M., Runyon, D.K., Edelsohn, G.A. and Coulter, M.L. (1989) 'Maternal support following disclosure of incest', *American Journal of Orthopsychiatry*, 59, 2: 197–207.

Fairtlough, A. (1983) *Responsibility for Incest: A Feminist View*, Norwich: Social Work Monograph, University of East Anglia.

Faller, K.C. (1988a) 'The myth of the "collusive mother": variability in the functioning of mothers of victims of intrafamilial sexual abuse', *Journal of Interpersonal Violence*, 3, 2: 190–6.

Faller, K.C. (1988b) *Child Sexual Abuse: An Interdisciplinary Manual for Diagnosis, Case Management and Treatment*, London: Macmillan Education.

Faller, K.C. (1989) 'Why sexual abuse? An exploration of the intergenerational hypothesis', *Child Abuse and Neglect*, 13: 543–9.

Ferraro, K. and Johnson, J. (1983) 'How women experience battering: the process of victimization', *Social Problems*, 30, 3: 325–9.

Ferraro, K.J. (1988) 'An existential approach to battering', in G.T. Hotaling *et al.* (eds), *Family Abuse and its Consequences: New Directions in Research*, London: Sage.

Finch, J. (1989) *Family Obligations and Social Change*, Cambridge: Polity.

Finkelhor, D. (1979) *Sexually Victimized Children*, New York: The Free Press.

Finkelhor, D. (1984) *Child Sexual Abuse: New Theory and Research*, New York: The Free Press.

Finkelhor, D. (1986a) *A Sourcebook on Child Sexual Abuse*, London: Sage.

Finkelhor, D. (1986b) 'Prevention approaches to child sexual abuse', in M. Lystad (ed.), *Violence in the Home: Interdisciplinary Perspectives*, New York: Brunner/ Mazel.

Finkelhor, D. and Browne, A. (1988) 'Assessing the long-term impact of child sexual abuse: a review and conceptualisation', in L. Walker (ed.), *Handbook on Sexual Abuse of Children*, New York: Springer.

Finkelhor, D. and Redfield, D. (1984) 'How the public defines sexual abuse', in D. Finkelhor (ed.), *Child Sexual Abuse: New Theory and Research*, New York: The Free Press.

Finkelhor, D. and Russell, D. (1984), 'Women as perpetrators: review of the evidence', in D. Finkelhor (ed.), *Child Sexual Abuse: New Theory and Research*, New York: The Free Press.

Freeman, M.D.A. (1983) *The Rights and Wrongs of Children*, London: Frances Pinter.

Frosh, S. (1988) 'No man's land? The role of men working with sexually abused children', *British Journal of Guidance and Counselling*, 16, 3: 1–10.

Frost, N. (1990) 'Official intervention and child protection: the relationship between state and family in contemporary Britain', in The Violence Against Children Study Group, *Taking Child Abuse Seriously*, London: Unwin Hyman.

Frost, N. and Stein, M. (1989) *The Politics of Child Welfare: Inequality, Power and Change*, Hemel Hempstead: Harvester Wheatsheaf.

Furniss, T. (1991) *The Multi-Professional Handbook of Child Sexual Abuse: Integrated Management, Therapy and Legal Intervention*, London: Routledge.

Gelles, R.J. (1976) 'Abused wives: why do they stay?', *Journal of Marriage and the Family*, 38, 4: 659–68.

Gershenson, H.P., Musick, J.S., Ruch-Ross, H.S., Magee, V., Rubino, K.K. and Rosenberg, D. (1989) 'The prevalence of coercive sexual experience among teenage mothers', *Journal of Interpersonal Violence*, 4, 2: 204–19.

Giddens, A. (1979) *Central Problems in Social Theory*, London: Macmillan.

Gilligan, C. (1982) *In a Different Voice: Psychological Theory and Women's Development*, Cambridge, Mass.: Harvard University Press.

Glaser, D. and Frosh, S. (1988) *Child Sexual Abuse*, London: Macmillan Education.

Glaser, D. and Spencer, J.R. (1990) 'Sentencing, children's evidence and children's trauma', *Criminal Law Review*, June: 371–82.

Glaser, B.G. and Straus, A.L. (1964) 'Awareness contexts and social interaction', *American Sociological Review*, 29, 5: 669–79.

Gomes-Schwartz, B., Horowitz, J.M. and Cardarelli, A.P. (1990) *Child Sexual Abuse: The Initial Effects*, London: Sage.

Goodwin, J. (1981) 'Suicide attempts in sexual abuse victims and their mothers', *Child Abuse and Neglect*, 5: 217–21.

Goodwin, J., McCarthy, T. and DiVasto, P. (1981) 'Prior incest in mothers of abused children', *Child Abuse and Neglect*, 5, 2: 87–95.

Gordon, L. (1986) 'Feminism and social control: the case of child abuse and neglect', in J. Mitchell and A. Oakley (eds), *What is Feminism?*, Oxford: Basil Blackwell.

Gordon, L. (1989) *Heroes of Their Own Lives: The Politics and History of Family Violence*, London: Virago.

Graham, D.L.R., Rawlings, E. and Rimini, N. (1988) 'Survivors of terror: battered women, hostages, and the Stockholm syndrome', in K. Yllo and M. Bograd (eds), *Feminist Perspectives on Wife Abuse*, London: Sage.

Graham, H. (1977) 'Women's attitudes to conception and pregnancy', in R. Chester and J. Peel (eds), *Equalities and Inequalities in Family Life*, London: Academic Press.

Graham, H. (1982) 'Coping: or how mothers are seen and not heard', in S. Friedman and E. Sarah (eds), *On the Problem of Men*, London: The Women's Press.

Graham, H. (1983) 'Caring: a labour of love', in J. Finch and D. Groves (eds), *A Labour of Love: Women, Work and Caring*, London: Routledge and Kegan Paul.

Graham, H. (1984) 'Surveying through stories', in C. Bell and H. Roberts (eds), *Social Researching: Politics, Problems, Practice*, London: Routledge and Kegan Paul.

Graham, H. (1985) 'Providers, negotiators and mediators: women as the hidden carers', in E. Lewin and V. Olesen (eds), *Women, Health and Healing*, London: Tavistock.

Greenwich Directorate of Social Services (1986) *Parent Participation in Child Abuse Review Conferences*, London Borough of Greenwich: Planning and Research Dept.

Hare-Mustin, R.T. (1987) 'The problem of gender in family therapy theory', *Family Process*, 26, 1: 15–28.

Herman, J. (1988) 'Considering sex offenders: a model of addiction', *Signs*, 13, 4: 695–724.

Herman, J. and Hirschman, L. (1977) 'Father–daughter incest', *Signs*, 2, 4: 735–56.

Herman, J. and Hirschman, L. (1981a) 'Families at risk for father–daughter incest', *American Journal of Psychiatry*, 138, 7: 967–70.

Herman, J.L. and Hirschman, L. (1981b), *Father–Daughter Incest*, Cambridge, Mass.: Harvard University Press.

Herzberger, S.D. and Tennen, H. (1988) 'Applying the label of physical abuse', in G.T. Hotaling *et al.* (eds), *Coping with Family Violence: Research and Policy Perspectives*, London: Sage.

Hildebrand, J. (1989) 'Group work with mothers of sexually abused children', in W.S. Rogers *et al.* (eds), *Child Abuse and Neglect*, London: Batsford.

Hildebrand, J. and Forbes, C. (1987) 'Group work with mothers whose children have been sexually abused', *British Journal of Social Work*, 17: 285–304.

Hoff, L.A. (1990) *Battered Women as Survivors*, London: Routledge.

Hooper, C.A. (1987) 'Getting him off the hook: the theory and practice of mother-blaming in child sexual abuse', *Trouble and Strife*, 12: 20–5.

Hooper, C.A. (1989a) 'Alternatives to collusion: the responses of mothers to child sexual abuse in the family', *Educational and Child Psychology*, 6, 1: 22–30.

Hooper, C.A (1989b) 'Rethinking the politics of child abuse', *Social History of Medicine*, 2, 3: 356–64.

Hooper, C.A. (1990) 'A study of mothers' responses to child sexual abuse by another family member'. Unpublished PhD thesis, University of London.

Hooper, C.A. (1992) 'Child sexual abuse and the regulation of women: variations on a theme', in C. Smart (ed.), *Regulating Womanhood*, London: Routledge.

Hopkins, J. and Thompson, E.H. (1984) 'Loss and mourning in victims of rape and sexual assault', in J. Hopkins (ed.), *Perspectives on Rape and Sexual Assault*, London: Harper and Row.

Hubbard, G.B. (1989) 'Mothers' perceptions of incest: sustained disruption and turmoil', *Archives of Psychiatric Nursing*, III, 1: 34–40.

Jacobs, J.L. (1990) 'Reassessing mother blame in incest', *Signs*, Spring: 500–14.

Janoff-Bulman, R. and Frieze, H. (1983) 'A theoretical perspective for understanding reactions to victimization', *Journal of Social Issues*, 39, 2: 1–17.

Johnson, B.K. and Kenkel, M.B. (1991) 'Stress, coping and adjustment in female adolescent incest victims', *Child Abuse and Neglect*, 15: 293–305.

Johnson, J.T. (1985) *An Ethnographic Study of Mothers in Father–Daughter Incest Families*, University of Pennsylvania: DSW thesis.

Johnson, M.M. (1982) 'Fathers and "femininity" in daughters: a review of the research', *Sociology and Social Research*, 67, 1: 1–17.

Johnson, M.M. (1988) *Strong Mothers, Weak Wives*, Berkeley: University of California Press.

Jones, D.P.H. (1991) 'Interviewing children', in K. Murray and D. Gough (eds), *Intervening in Child Sexual Abuse*, Edinburgh: Scottish Academic Press.

Jones, D., Pickett, J., Oates, M.R. and Barbor, P.R.H. (1987) *Understanding Child Abuse*, Basingstoke: Macmillan.

Jones, S. (1985a) 'Depth interviewing', in R. Walker (ed.), *Applied Qualitative Research*, Aldershot: Gower.

Jones, S. (1985b) 'The analysis of depth interviews', in R. Walker (ed.), *Applied Qualitative Research*, Aldershot: Gower.

Joshi, H. (1987) 'The cost of caring', in C. Glendinning and J. Millar (eds), *Women and Poverty in Britain*, Brighton: Wheatsheaf.

Kadushin, A. and Martin, J.A. (1981) *Child Abuse, an Interactional Event*, New York: Columbia University Press.

Kalichman, S.C., Craig, M.E. and Follingstad, D.R. (1990) 'Professionals' adherence to mandatory child abuse reporting laws: effects of responsibility attribution, confidence ratings and situational factors', *Child Abuse and Neglect*, 14: 69–77.

Kaufman, I., Peck, A.L. and Tagiuri, C.I. (1954) 'The family constellation and overt incestuous relations between father and daughter', *American Journal of Orthopsychiatry*, 24: 266–78.

Kelley, S.J. (1990) 'Parental stress response to sexual abuse and ritualistic abuse of children in day-care centers', *Nursing Research*, 39, 1: 25–9.

Kelly, L. (1988a) *Surviving Sexual Violence*, Cambridge: Polity.

Kelly, L. (1988b) 'What's in a name? Defining child sexual abuse', *Feminist Review*, 28: 65–73.

Kelly, L. (1988c) 'How women define their experiences of violence', in K. Yllo and M. Bograd (eds), *Feminist Perspectives on Wife Abuse*, London: Sage.

Kelly, L. (1989) 'Bitter ironies: the professionalisation of child sexual abuse', *Trouble and Strife*, 16: 14–21.

Kelly, L. (1991) 'Unspeakable acts: women who abuse', *Trouble and Strife*, 21: 13–20.

Kelly, L., Regan, L. and Burton, S. (1991) *An Exploratory Study of the Prevalence of Sexual Abuse in a Sample of 16–21 Year Olds*, Polytechnic of North London: Child Abuse Studies Unit.

Kempe, R.S. and Kempe, C.H. (1978) *Child Abuse*, London: Fontana/Open Books.

Kirkwood, C.M. (1991) 'From the scars of survival to wisdom for change: the experiences of formerly abused women'. Unpublished PhD thesis, University of York.

Koss, M., Gidycz, C. and Wisniewski, N. (1987) 'The scope of rape: incidence and prevalence of sexual aggression in a national sample of higher education students', *Journal of Consulting and Clinical Psychology*, 55: 162–70.

La Fontaine, J. (1990) *Child Sexual Abuse*, Cambridge: Polity.

Lane, S. (1986) 'Women and child care: factors influencing social work dealings in women's lives', *British Journal of Social Work*, 16: 111–23.

Leiulfsrud, H. and Woodward, A.E. (1988) 'Women at class crossroads: a critical reply to Erikson and Goldthorpe's Note', *Sociology*, 22, 4: 555–62.

Leroi, D.E. (1984) *The Silent Partner: an Investigation of the Familial*

Background, Personality Structure, Sexual Behaviour and Relationships of the Mothers of Incestuous Families, University of Berkeley, California: PhD thesis.

Levang, C.A. (1988) 'Interactional communication patterns in father/daughter incest families', *Journal of Psychology and Human Sexuality*, 1, 2: 53–68.

Lewis, J. and Meredith, B. (1988) *Daughters Who Care*, London: Routledge.

Lisak, D. (1991) 'Sexual aggression, masculinity and fathers', *Signs*, 16, 2: 238–62.

London Borough of Brent (1985) *A Child in Trust: Report of the Panel of Inquiry Investigating the Circumstances Surrounding the Death of Jasmine Beckford*, London Borough of Brent.

London Borough of Greenwich (1987) *A Child in Mind: Protection of Children in a Responsible Society, The Report of the Commission of Inquiry into the Circumstances Surrounding the Death of Kimberley Carlile*, London Borough of Greenwich.

London Borough of Lambeth (1987) *Whose Child? A Report of the Public Inquiry into the Death of Tyra Henry*, London Borough of Lambeth.

Luker, K. (1975) *Taking Chances: Abortion and the Decision not to Contracept*, Berkeley: University of California Press.

Lustig, N., Dresser, J.W., Spellman, S.W. and Murray, T.B. (1966) 'Incest, a family group survival pattern', *Archives of General Psychiatry*, 14: 31–40.

McGibbon, A., Cooper, L. and Kelly, L. (1989) *What Support? An Exploratory Study of Council Policy and Practice, and Local Support Services in the Area of Domestic Violence within Hammersmith and Fulham*, Polytechnic of North London: Child Abuse Studies Unit.

McGovern, K. and Peters, J. (1988) 'Guidelines for assessing sex offenders', in L. Walker (ed.), *Handbook on Sexual Abuse of Children*, New York: Springer.

MacLeod, M. and Saraga, E. (1988) 'Challenging the orthodoxy: towards a feminist theory and practice', *Feminist Review*, 28: 16–55.

MacLeod, M. and Saraga, E. (1991) 'Clearing a path through the undergrowth: a feminist reading of recent literature on child sexual abuse', in P. Carter *et al.* (eds), *Social Work and Social Welfare Yearbook 3*, Milton Keynes: Open University Press.

Mama, A. (1989) *The Hidden Struggle: Statutory and Voluntary Responses to Violence against Black Women in the Home*, London: London Race and Housing Research Unit.

Manchershaw, A. (1987) *A Study of Sexual Abuse in Women Attending a General Practice: Prevalence, Disclosure and Psychological Adjustment*, British Psychological Society Diploma in Clinical Psychology: Research dissertation.

Markowe, L. (1990) *The Coming-Out Process for Lesbians*, University of London: PhD thesis.

Marris, P. (1986) *Loss and Change*, London: Routledge and Kegan Paul.

Marsden, D. and Abrams, S. (1987) '"Liberators", "companions", "intruders" and "cuckoos in the nest": a sociology of caring relationships over the life cycle', in P. Allatt *et al.* (eds), *Women and The Life Cycle*, Basingstoke: Macmillan.

Masson, H. and O'Byrne, P. (1990) 'The family systems approach: a help or a hindrance?', in The Violence Against Children Study Group, *Taking Child Abuse Seriously*, London: Unwin Hyman.

Mayer, J.E. and Timms, N. (1970) *The Client Speaks: Working Class Impressions of Casework*, London: Routledge and Kegan Paul.

Maynard, M. (1985) 'The response of social workers to domestic violence', in J. Pahl (ed.), *Private Violence and Public Policy: The Needs of Battered Women and the Response of Public Services*, London: Routledge and Kegan Paul.

Metropolitan Police and Bexley Social Services (1987) *Child Sexual Abuse Joint Investigative Programme, Bexley Experiment*, London: HMSO.

Millar, J. (1987) 'Lone mothers', in C. Glendinning and J. Millar (eds), *Women and Poverty in Britain*, Brighton: Wheatsheaf.

Miller, A.C. (1990) 'The mother–daughter relationship and the distortion of reality in childhood sexual abuse', in R.J. Perelberg and A.C. Miller (eds), *Gender and Power in Families*, London: Routledge.

Mitchell, C.J. (1983) 'Case and situation analysis', *The Sociological Review*, 31, 2: 187–211.

Mitra, C. (1987) 'Judicial discourse in father–daughter incest appeal cases', *International Journal of the Sociology of Law*, 15, 2: 121–48.

Muller, A. (1987) *Parents Matter: Parents' Relationships with Lesbian Daughters and Gay Sons*, Tallahassee, Florida: The Naiad Press.

Myer, M. (1984) 'A new look at mothers of incest victims', *Journal of Social Work and Human Sexuality*, 3: 47–58.

Nelson, S. (1987) *Incest: Fact and Myth*, Edinburgh: Stramullion Press, 2nd edn.

O'Hagan, K. (1989) *Working with Child Sexual Abuse*, Milton Keynes: Open University Press.

Oliver, M. (1983) *Social Work with Disabled People*, Basingstoke: Macmillan.

Ong, B.N. (1985) 'The paradox of wonderful children: the case of child abuse', *Early Child Development and Care*, 21: 91–106.

Packman, J. and Randall, J. (1989) 'Decision-making at the gateway to care', in O. Stevenson (ed.), *Child Abuse: Public Policy and Professional Practice*, Hemel Hempstead: Harvester Wheatsheaf.

Pahl, J. (ed.) (1985) *Private Violence and Public Policy: The Needs of Battered Women and the Response of the Public Services*, London: Routledge and Kegan Paul.

Pahl, J. (1989) *Money and Marriage*, London: Macmillan.

Parton, C. (1990) 'Women, gender oppression and child abuse', in The Violence Against Children Study Group, *Taking Child Abuse Seriously*, London: Unwin Hyman.

Parton, C. and Parton, N. (1988/9) 'Women, the family and child protection', *Critical Social Policy*, 24: 38–49.

Parton, C. and Parton, N. (1989) 'Child protection, the law and dangerousness', in O. Stevenson (ed.), *Child Abuse: Public Policy and Professional Practice*, Hemel Hempstead: Harvester Wheatsheaf.

Parton, N. (1991) *Governing the Family: Child Care, Child Protection and the State*, London: Macmillan.

Parton, N. and Martin, N. (1989) 'Public inquiries, legalism and child care in England and Wales', *International Journal of Law and the Family*, 3, 1: 21–39.

Parton, N. and Small, N. (1989) 'Violence, social work and the emergence of dangerousness', in M. Langan and P. Lee (eds), *Radical Social Work Today*, London: Unwin Hyman.

Pateman, C. (1985) *The Problem of Political Obligation*, Cambridge: Polity.

Pateman, C. (1988) *The Sexual Contract*, Cambridge: Polity.

Peace, G. and McMaster, J. (1989) *Child Sexual Abuse: Professional and Personal Perspectives Part 1: Aspects of Investigation*, Cheadle: The Boys and Girls Welfare Society.

Pellegrin, A. and Wagner, W.G. (1990) 'Child sexual abuse: factors affecting victims' removal from home', *Child Abuse and Neglect*, 14: 53–60.

Phoenix, A. (1991) *Young Mothers?*, Cambridge: Polity.

Pigot Committee (1989) *Report of the Advisory Group on Video Evidence*, London: Home Office.

Pithouse, A. (1987) *Social Work: The Social Organisation of an Invisible Trade*, Aldershot: Avebury.

Potter, J. and Wetherell, M. (1987) *Discourse and Social Psychology*, London: Sage.

Pringle, K. (1990) *Managing to Survive: Developing a Resource for Sexually Abused Young People*, Family Placement Project, Barnardos North East.

Raphael-Leff, T. (1983) 'Facilitators and regulators: two approaches to mothering', *British Journal of Medical Psychology*, 56: 379–90.

Regehr, C. (1990) 'Parental responses to extrafamilial child sexual abuse', *Child Abuse and Neglect*, 14: 113–20.

Reid, C. (1989) *Mothers of Sexually Abused Girls: A Feminist View*, Norwich: Social Work Monograph, University of East Anglia.

Remer, R. and Elliott, J.E. (1988a) 'Characteristics of secondary victims of sexual assault', *International Journal of Psychiatry*, 9, 4: 373–87.

Remer, R. and Elliott, J.E. (1988b) 'Management of secondary victims of sexual assault', *International Journal of Psychiatry*, 9, 4: 389–401.

Ribbens, J. (1990) 'Accounting for our Children: Differing Perspectives on 'Family Life' in Middle-Income Households'. Unpublished PhD thesis, South Bank Polytechnic, London.

Rich, A. (1977) *Of Woman Born: Motherhood as Experience and Institution*, London: Virago.

Ringwalt, C. and Earp, J. (1988) 'Attributing responsibility – cases of father–daughter sexual abuse', *Child Abuse and Neglect*, 12: 273–81.

Roberts, C.M. (1988) *A Summary of: A Review of Good Practice in the Treatment of Child Sexual Abuse*, Report for a Working Party of the Borough Review Committee, London Borough of Wandsworth.

Runyan, D.K. *et al.* (1988) 'Impact of legal intervention on sexually abused children', *The Journal of Paediatrics*, 113, 4: 647–53.

Russell, D. (1984) *Sexual Exploitation: Rape, Child Sexual Abuse and Workplace Harassment*, London: Sage.

Ryan, T.S. (1986) 'Problems, errors and opportunities in the treatment of father–daughter incest', *Journal of Interpersonal Violence*, 1, 1: 113–24.

Sapiro, V. (1990) 'The gender basis of American social policy', in L. Gordon (ed.), *Women, the State and Welfare*, Wisconsin: University of Wisconsin Press.

Schatzow, E. and Herman, J. (1989) 'Breaking secrecy: adult survivors disclose to their families', *Psychiatric Clinics of North America*, 12, 2: 337–49.

SCOSAC (1984) *Definition of Child Sexual Abuse*, London: Standing Committee on Sexually Abused Children, London.

Scott, J.W. (1988) *Gender and the Politics of History*, New York: Columbia University Press.

Scott, R.S. and Flowers, J.V. (1988) 'Betrayal by the mother as a factor contributing to psychological disturbance in victims of father–daughter incest: an MMPI analysis', *Journal of Social and Clinical Psychology*, 6, 1: 147–54.

Scutt, J.A. (1988) 'The privatisation of justice: power differentials, inequality and the palliative of counselling and mediation', *Women's Studies International Forum*, 11, 5: 503–20.

Secretary of State for Social Services (1988) *Report of the Inquiry into Child Abuse in Cleveland 1987*, London: HMSO.

Sedlak, A.J. (1988) 'The effects of personal experiences with couple violence on calling it "battering" and allocating blame', in G.T. Hotaling *et al.* (eds), *Coping with Family Violence: Research and Policy Perspectives*, London: Sage.

Sgroi, S.M. (1982) *Handbook of Clinical Intervention in Child Sexual Abuse*, Lexington, Mass: Lexington Books.

Shemmings, D. and Thoburn, J. (1990) *Parental Participation in Child Protection Conferences: Report of a Pilot Project in Hackney Social Services Department*, Norwich: Social Work Development Unit, University of East Anglia.

Shields, N.M. and Hanneke, C.R. (1988) 'Multiple sexual victimization: the case of incest and marital rape', in G.T. Hotaling *et al.* (eds), *Coping with Family Violence: Research and Policy Perspectives*, London: Sage.

Sirles, E.A. and Franke, P.J. (1989) 'Factors influencing mothers' reactions to intrafamily sexual abuse', *Child Abuse and Neglect*, 13, 1: 131–9.

Sirles, E.A. and Lofberg, C.E. (1990) 'Factors associated with divorce in intrafamily child sexual abuse cases', *Child Abuse and Neglect*, 14: 165–70.

Sloane, P. and Karpinski, E. (1942) 'Effects of incest on the participants', *American Journal of Orthopsychiatry*, 12: 666–73.

Smart, C. (1989) *Feminism and the Power of Law*, London: Routledge.

Stark, E. and Flitcraft, A. (1983) 'Social knowledge, social policy, and the abuse of women: the case against patriarchal benevolence', in D. Finkelhor (ed.), *The Dark Side of Families*, Beverly Hills, California: Sage.

Stark, E. and Flitcraft, A. (1988) 'Women and children at risk: a feminist perspective on child abuse', *International Journal of Health Services*, 18, 1: 97–118.

Stevenson, O. (ed.) (1989a) *Child Abuse: Public Policy and Professional Practice*, Hemel Hempstead: Harvester Wheatsheaf.

Stevenson, O. (1989b) 'Reflections on social work practice', in O. Stevenson (ed.), *Child Abuse: Public Policy and Professional Practice*, Hemel Hempstead: Harvester Wheatsheaf.

Straus, A.L. (1987) *Qualitative Analysis for Social Scientists*, Cambridge: Cambridge University Press.

Strube, M.J. (1988) 'The decision to leave an abusive relationship: empirical evidence and theoretical issues', *Psychological Bulletin*, 104, 2: 236–50.

Strube, M.J. and Barbour, L.S. (1983) 'The decision to leave an abusive relationship: economic dependence and psychological commitment', *Journal of Marriage and the Family*, 45, 4: 785–94.

Summit, R. (1983) 'The child sexual abuse accommodation syndrome', *Child Abuse and Neglect*, 7: 177–94.

Summit, R. (1988) 'Hidden victims, hidden pain: societal avoidance of child sexual abuse', in G.E. Wyatt and G.J. Powell (eds), *Lasting Effects of Child Sexual Abuse*, London: Sage.

Thoennes, N. and Tjaden, P.G. (1990) 'The extent, nature and validity of sexual abuse allegations in custody/visitation disputes', *Child Abuse and Neglect*, 14: 151–63.

Thornes, B. and Collard, J. (1979) *Who Divorces?*, London: Routledge and Kegan Paul.

Truesdell, D.J., McNeil, J.S. and Deschner, J.P. (1986) 'Incidence of wife abuse in incestuous families', *Social Work*, March–April: 138–40.

Turner, S.F. and Shapiro, C.H. (1986) 'Battered women: mourning the death of a relationship', *Social Work*, 31, 5: 372–6.

Ungerson, C. (1987) *Policy is Personal: Sex, Gender and Informal Care*, London: Tavistock.

The Violence Against Children Study Group (1990) *Taking Child Abuse Seriously*, London: Unwin Hyman.

Vizard, E. and Tranter, M. (1988) 'Recognition and assessment of child sexual abuse', in A. Bentovim *et al.* (eds), *Child Sexual Abuse within the Family: Assessment and Treatment*, London: Wright.

Wagner, W.G. (1991) 'Depression in mothers of sexually abused children vs mothers of non-abused children', *Child Abuse and Neglect*, 15: 99–104.

Walker, L. (ed.) (1988) *Handbook on Sexual Abuse of Children: Assessment and Treatment Issues*, New York: Springer.

Walkerdine, V. and Lucey, H. (1989) *Democracy in the Kitchen: Regulating Mothers and Socialising Daughters*, London: Virago Press.

Ward, E. (1984) *Father–Daughter Rape*, London: The Women's Press.

Wattam, C. *et al.* (1989) *Child Sexual Abuse*, Harlow: Longman.

Wattenberg, E. (1985) 'In a different light: a feminist perspective on the role of mothers in father–daughter incest', *Child Welfare*, LXIV, 3: 203–11.

Widom, C.S. (1989) 'The cycle of violence', *UM Science*, 244, 4901: 160–6.

Wilczynski, A. (1991) 'Neonaticide'. Paper presented at the 'Perspectives on Female Violence' National Conference, St George's Hospital Medical School, London, 7–8 March 1991.

Wilk, R.J. and McCarthy, C.R. (1986) 'Intervention in child sexual abuse: a survey of attitudes', *Social Casework*, 67, 1: 20–6.

Willmott, P. (1986) *Social Networks, Informal Care and Public Policy*, Research Report 655, Policy Studies Institute, London.

Women's Research Centre (1989) *Recollecting our Lives: Women's Experiences of Childhood Sexual Abuse*, Vancouver: Press Gang Publishers.

Woodcraft, E. (1988) 'Child sexual abuse and the law', *Feminist Review*, 28: 122–30.

Wootton, B. (1959) *Social Science and Social Pathology*, London: Routledge and Kegan Paul.

Wright, E. and Portnoy, S. (1990) 'Helping mothers in crisis', *Community Care*, 25.1.90: 22–3.

Wyatt, G.E. and Mickey, M.R. (1987) 'Ameliorating the effects of child sexual abuse: an exploratory study of support by parents and others', *Journal of Interpersonal Violence*, 2, 4: 403–14.

Wyatt, G.E and Newcomb, M. (1990) 'Internal and external mediators of women's sexual abuse in childhood', *Journal of Consulting and Clinical Psychology*, 58, 6: 758–67.

Wyatt, G.E. and Powell, G.J. (eds) (1988) *Lasting Effects of Child Sexual Abuse*, London: Sage.

Yllo, K. and Bograd, M. (eds) (1988) *Feminist Perspectives on Wife Abuse*, London: Sage.

Zuravin, S.J. (1987) 'Unplanned pregnancies, family planning problems and child maltreatment', *Family Relations*, 36, 2: 135–9.

Index